Choose **WELL** ᴛᴏ Live **WELL**

THE FIVE FUNDAMENTALS TO CREATE A FIT, HEALTHY AND STRONG BODY AND MIND!

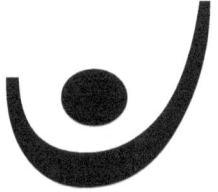

Lᴀᴜʀᴀ Bᴏɴɪᴇʟʟᴏ

The rise of a new day is a fresh start, a clean slate. What a gift! Choose well! You always have the power to choose.

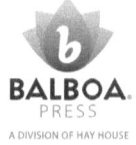

BALBOA
PRESS
A DIVISION OF HAY HOUSE

ISBN: 978-1-4525-6082-3(sc)
ISBN: 978-1-4525-6084-7(hc)
ISBN: 978-1-4525-6083-0(e)
Balboa Press books may be ordered through booksellers or by contacting:

Balboa Press
A Division of Hay House
1663 Liberty Drive
Bloomington, IN 47403
www.balboapress.com
1-(877) 407-4847

Library of Congress Control Number: 2012920170
Printed in the United States of America

Balboa Press rev. date: 10/22/2012

CONTENTS

PREFACE

Ready to get back to basics!

I TRULY BELIEVE THE purpose of life is to enjoy all aspects of your world, and it's tough to enjoy life if you're not well physically and emotionally and have continuous feelings of stress, worry, and anxiety. We are here to *experience life*. Why not experience it with a healthy body and a healthy mind? We have a huge amount of control over the health and wellness of our physical body and our state of mind. It all boils down to your *choices*. Life is all about making choices and experiencing the results of those choices. Conscious or not, we are responsible for every choice we make.

My intention with this book is to encourage and help you create a fit, strong, healthy body and state of mind, one choice at a time. The five steps are fundamental practices that, when repeated, become healthy habits. Healthy habits create a healthy lifestyle. A healthy lifestyle creates the fit, strong, healthy body and state of mind you want to experience your life through.

Choose Well to Live Well is a *lifestyle* that needs to be *practiced and lived* one day at a time. This is really about bringing *awareness* to the choices you have been making up to this point and the results of those choices. It's about learning to tweak your choices in order to experience a healthier, happier life. It's about making little changes—one day, one choice at a time. You can always tweak and change something, whether it's your attitude, your food choices, who you spend your time with, or what you put your attention on. These small tweaks add up to healthy changes over a period of time. The dictionary defines lifestyle as "the habits, attitude, tastes, etc., that together constitute the mode of living of an individual or group." *Choose Well to Live Well* offers a way of living. Commit to living the *Choose Well to Live Well* five fundamentals every day and enjoy the benefits of reaping a fit, strong, healthy body and state of mind!

INTRODUCTION

THERE IS POWER in owning your choices and taking responsibility for everything showing up in your life. Own that power. Every healthy change begins with a choice. You have the power within you right here and right now to live a healthier and happier life no matter what you're experiencing right now. This lifestyle program is meant to help *you* figure out what is best for *you*. What works well for one person may not be the best for you. Choosing well to live well is about taking responsibility for everything you're experiencing and tweaking or changing specific choices in order to reap a better result. It's about figuring out what's best for you to create the life and health you want to experience.

Everyone can benefit from a peaceful and calm state of mind. I have had the pleasure of working with clients for more than twenty years in the fitness and wellness field, and I have taught these basics and live them myself. I am thrilled to share these basics to help *you* live a healthy and happy life, as I have with many clients. The best part about practicing your basics is the amazing way life unfolds for you. Once you become conscious of your choices and start deliberately choosing the five basics, you will be amazed where the journey can take you. Once you start feeling healthy, fit, and strong in both mind and body, life unfolds for you in an incredible way.

This lifestyle program is also intended to help you become aware of and avoid what I call a "toxic cycle." What is a toxic cycle? It's when you allow yourself to get into unhealthy patterns that cause toxins to build up in your body, which makes you susceptible to illness and disease. There is always something you can do for your health and well-being. And not doing anything to improve your health enables a toxic cycle. For example, people often work a tremendous amount of hours during the week. Since they're working so much, they're too exhausted to get up for a workout. Since they're too exhausted to get up for a workout, they don't feel well. They then start eating like crap and drink too much coffee and not enough water, which makes their body and mind feel worse. Since they don't feel well, their mood is down, and everything that happens during the day is emotionally worse for them because they don't feel well in the first place. You may find yourself getting angry, frustrated, and impatient very easily if you haven't moved your body to release stress and tension from it, ate junk food, didn't get enough sleep, and are dehydrated. This is a "toxic cycle." Although the five fundamentals are recommended to work together, if you commit to just one or two at a time, *you will start to feel healthier and better!*

It is my hope, prayer, and intention that this lifestyle program will help you live a healthy, fit, and happy life. That this simple program will help you go from a victim (a victim of yourself and your circumstances) to a creator and will awaken within you the fact that you really do have the power to create everything you experience in your world. That you will practice these healthy habits, make them your personal way of living, and avoid a toxic cycle. You can take control of your life, your health, and your happiness by deliberately taking control of the choices you are making—one day, one step at a time.

I would recommend you approach this book as a personal health and wellness coaching manual. It's your personal journey to better health and well-being. You take the steps by making the choices that are best for you right now tweaking and adjusting as you go along, using this book as a guide. This is how I coach clients to better health and well-being, and I am thrilled to share it with you!

Thank you for allowing me to be a part of your health and wellness journey.

Enjoy your journey, enjoy your "practice," and enjoy how your life unfolds. I wish you peace, calmness, abundance, and brilliant health and happiness.

Please visit www.choosewelltolivewell.com for more support in living the Choose Well lifestyle!

To get through the hardest journey, we need take only one step at a time, but we must keep on stepping.
—Chinese Proverb

To keep the body in good health is our duty; otherwise we shall not be able to keep our mind strong and clear.
—Buddha

CHOOSE WELL TO LIVE
WELL CONCEPTS

L IFE IS ABOUT **making choices.**

We are each responsible for the choices we make; hence we are each responsible for our life.

Every thought we choose to think, every word we choose to say, every action we choose to take, and every attitude we choose to give creates our experiences.

Live and choose now. Now is all we have.

Everything is energy. You "give" your world your chosen energy in the form of what you think, what you say, what you do, and the attitude you bring to yourself, those around you, and all aspects of your life. What you give your world is what you receive back from it, and you are always giving.

You will attract the same energy that you give away. What are you giving?

Every choice reaps a result and consequence. The universal law of cause and effect is at work all the time. Every choice matters. Every choice counts.

When you change and tweak your choices, you change your experiences and circumstances.

You choose to live your life either from a place of love or from a place of fear. What are you choosing? What will you choose? Are you looking at life through the eyes of love or the eyes of fear? Life unfolds very differently based on this choice.

You always have the power of choice. Own it. If you don't own it, you will be swayed and influenced by other people and circumstances around you.

Our lives are fashioned by our choices.
First we make our choices. Then our choices make us.
—Anne Frank

Choose-Well Lifestyle Questions

I'M SURE YOU heard the saying "the definition of insanity is doing the same thing repeatedly and expecting a different result." How true. I also believe that insanity is "being" the same thing repeatedly and expecting a different result. In other words, bring the same negative attitude with you through your day, and nothing will change for the better. Spend your time and energy on circumstances and people that drain you, and you will feel drained, exhausted, and sick. You need to bring an attitude and action that result in a positive change in order to experience something different. All change begins with you. It takes an open mind and a willing heart to dig in deep and really take a look at what you're choosing *to do and be*, and where you're putting your energy and attention.

Let's take a snapshot look at what you're choosing to be and do right now in your life by answering a series of questions. In order to make positive and healthy changes in your life, you need to bring some awareness of what's happening and what you're choosing right now.

If you love what you're living and experiencing, keep choosing the same thoughts, attitudes, and behavior. If you don't love an area of your life, it's up to you to look in the mirror and change/tweak what you need to in your thoughts, attitude, and behavior in order to experience a better result. Changing things outside of you may seem easier, but it's exhausting and energy-draining. It's actually a lot harder to manipulate the external circumstances. One tweak in how you think, in your attitude and behavior, can cause a huge shift in the results you're experiencing.

Answer honestly, with no judgment or analyzing. This is not a time for excuses, blaming, and justifying why you're making the choices you're making. It's just a time to take a snapshot of what *you* are doing and being. This is not a time for guilt, frustration, or feeling angry at yourself. The purpose of answering these questions is to *bring awareness to what you're choosing and experiencing up to this point in your life so you can make positive changes by choosing better.* You will learn so much about yourself and your life by just answering these questions! You have to be aware and wake up to what you are choosing in order to make changes.

How's life?

What's working really well for you?

What's not quite working as well as you would like it to?

Why do you think that is?

How much do you weigh? Do you feel healthy at this weight? How much do you need to lose/gain in order to feel healthy and well?

What is your clothes size? What do you want your clothes size to be?

Are you married or do you have a significant other? Children? Pets?

What's your occupation? How many hours do you work (include commute time) per week?

Do you enjoy what you do for a living?

What is your stress level, 1 being not feeling stressed, and 10 being feeling highly stressed?

What is the main source of your stress right now?

Is there anything you do right now to relieve your stress?

Do you smoke?

Do you take medications? If so, for what?

How do you feel most of the time? (Happy, at ease, content, stressed, anxious, worried, calm …?)

Sleep

How many hours do you sleep? How many hours of sleep do you need to feel well?

Do you go to bed at the same time and
wake up at the same time daily?

Do you sleep well?

Do you wake up frequently?

Are you energized upon rising?

Do you exercise consistently?

Do you drink alcohol at night? How much?

Do you drink coffee or any caffeinated drinks?
How much? How late in the day?

How much water do you drink, and how late do you drink it?

What is your evening ritual or evening habits? List all activities you
engage in before sleep. (Read? TV? Computer? Work? Meditate?)

What time is your last meal at night?

What is your typical dinner?

Do you snack at night?

What relaxes you? What calms your mind down?

Do you pray? Do you journal? Do you meditate?

Action Step: Taking a look at your answers above.
What can you choose to start doing in
order to get a better quality sleep?

Is there anything you need to stop doing to get a better quality sleep?

What attitude do you need to practice to make this happen?

Food and Liquids

What are you eating? (Include breakfast, lunch, dinner, snacks.)

Are your meals home-cooked?

What time do you eat your meals?

How do you eat your meals? (Calm, sitting, and slow?
Or on the run, fast, and while doing other things?)

Any digestive issues?

Do you drink alcohol? When and how much?

Do you drink coffee? When and how much?

How much water do you drink a day?

Do you experience headaches?

Do you drink soda, diet soda, juice, or anything
sugary? .... When and how much?

Do you have any cravings? Food, alcohol, drugs, etc.?

Do you take vitamins or supplements? If so, what do you take?

How often do you eat fast food?

How often do you eat out?

Do you practice portion control?

What time of day do you eat your largest meal?

Do you feel you eat balanced meals? (carb/protein/fats at every meal)

Do you read food labels when shopping?

Do you buy organic? If yes, what?

Do you skip meals?

Are you preoccupied with food? Do you
think about food all the time?

Do you eat meat? What kind and how often?

Do you buy organic meat?

How many servings of fruits and vegetables are you getting per day?

Do you eat packaged/processed foods? How often?

Action Step: Look at your answers to the above questions.
What is one thing you can choose to start doing right now
that will make a healthy impact on your physical body and
your state of mind in regards to food and drink choices?
Is there something you need to stop choosing in
regards to food and drink choices to make a healthy
impact on your body and state of mind?
What attitude do you need to practice to make this happen?

Exercise/Hobby/Activities

Do you exercise? Where? When?

What do you do? How long? How often?

What activity did you enjoy growing up?

Is your activity and movement balanced? In other words, do you engage in cardio, strength and core conditioning, and flexibility exercises?

How does your physical body feel? Healthy, energized, and fit? Or tired, bloated, in pain and/or sick?

Are you in any physical pain? If yes, what are you doing about the pain?

Do you get outside in nature?

How often?

What activities do you enjoy? How often do you engage in these activities?

Do you have any hobbies that renew your spirit?

How often do you engage in these hobbies?

Action Step: Take a look at your answers above. What is one thing you can start doing today, in regards to movement and exercise, that will make a healthy impact on the wellness of your body and state of mind?

Is there a something you need to stop doing?

What attitude do you need to practice to make this happen?

Do you watch TV? How much per day? What type of show/movies?

Do you read? What do you read? How much do you read?

Do you watch the news or read the newspaper? When?..How much?

Do you meditate? Pray? Journal? Have a gratitude practice? Do breathing exercises? Go to church or spiritual practice? How often?

What connects you to your spirit? How often do
you engage in spirit-connecting activities?
Do you spend time alone in silence? How often?
Do you spend time outside in nature? How often?
How much time do you spend on social media? Do you find this
an uplifting nurturing experience? Do you find experiencing
social media stressful, time consuming, or distracting?
Do you use alternative natural healers?
Chiropractors, massage therapists, etc.?
How do you feel the majority of the time? (Calm,
stressed, anxious, energized, tired?)
Are the people you associate with uplifting, encouraging,
and positive? Or do you feel wiped out and exhausted
after spending time with them? Be specific and list the
relationships that nurture and uplift you, the ones that drain
your energy, and how much time you spend with them.

Managing Your State of Mind and Attitude

You are the center of all aspects of your life, the major ones being relationships, work/money/career, and the health of your physical body.

You bring your energy in the form of your attitude and mood, your thoughts and perceptions, your words and conversations, your action and behavior to each aspect of your life. Your thinking, saying, behavior, and attitude create your experience.

Everything you're living is the perfect result of the energy you're giving. If there's an area of your life that is not quite working as well as you would like, check in with the energy you're giving and the choices you've made up to this point. You can work your tail off, but without checking in with the attitude you're giving as you're working hard, you could be getting in your own way and not get the results you're looking for.

Let's take a look (without judgment, justifications, or excuses) at what *you* are "giving" right now.

Relationships

On a scale of 1–10, how nurturing, supportive, and loving are your relationships? Go ahead and list the most important people in your life and give the relationship a snapshot rating.

What attitude and energy have *you* been giving your relationships? Are your thoughts, conversations, behavior, and attitude nourishing, helpful, and uplifting? Or are they toxic, negative, and destructive?

How do you want your relationships to be?

However you want your relationships to be, you need to "be" that state first. If you want support, you need to be supportive. If you want peace, you need to be peaceful first. If you want love, you need to be loving. With that said, what energy can you start giving in the form of attitude to make the relationships around you better? (Love, kindness, patience, acceptance, appreciation?)

Physical Body

On a scale of 1–10, how is the health and fitness of your physical body?

Have you been taking care of your body? What is the most important thing you can do right now to take care of your body?

Is your attention and awareness on "wellness" or on "illness"?

What attitude and energy have you been giving your physical body? Appreciating? Or criticizing and complaining?

Now—right now—**vow to never criticize yourself or your physical body ever again**. Start embracing and loving your body, right now ... no matter what.

List everything you appreciate about your physical body. List everything that makes you smile about your body.

Work/Finances/Career

On a scale of 1–10, how fulfilling and satisfying is your career?

What attitude/energy have you been giving your work? Is it positive, uplifting, helpful, and nurturing? Or is it negative, fearful, worrying, toxic energy?

What are your conversations like? Are you speaking helpful, nourishing, positive, and uplifting words? Or are they negative, complaining, worrying, fearful conversations?

Are your associations encouraging, helpful, and uplifting? Or do they drag you down?

Does your work fulfill you?

Do you enjoy what you are doing?

Can you start enjoying it? Or do you need to go in a different direction?

Are you focused on the positives of your job/work or the negatives most of the time?

What is one thing you can start doing to make your work environment, financial situation, or career better?

What attitude can you bring to your work, finances, or business that will improve your experience?

List everything you appreciate about your current job, career, and finances. List what makes you smile about your work and career. If you are having a hard time with this, dig in deep and really focus on what you can be grateful for.

If you need to make a change of direction, what's one thing you can start doing to put yourself in the right direction that makes you feel good?

Happy List

What turns you on?

What do you love to do?

What recharges your batteries when you feel
overwhelmed, tired, and running on empty?
What makes you feel good?
What feeds your soul? What renews your spirit?
List everything that feeds your soul.

Take a look at how you answered the first question: how's life?
If your answer is anything less than good, exciting, amazing, joyful,
awesome, realize that life is bringing you exactly how you feel about
it.

What about the second question? Are you bringing a state of
appreciation to what's working well for you in your life? Are you
acknowledging the goodness or taking it for granted?

What about the third question? Are you blaming outside
circumstances and other people for what isn't working well for you
right now? If so, you're living in a victim mentality, and the only
way to make positive changes is to take your power back, take
responsibility for all that's going on in your life, and start making
healthier choices.

Choose well to live well!

My Story

LIFE IS AN amazing and incredible journey—full of highs and lows, ups and downs. I sometimes look back and think, *Wow, a lot has happened so far in my life.* It's as if we live many lives within one lifetime. The lows and challenges become opportunities for growth and strength. The highs are for pure enjoyment. All moments are meant to be experienced. I am going to share with you two of my life-changing experiences and what I learned from them.

If you're going through a tough time in any area of your life, I encourage you to dig in deep and look inside yourself to see how you're creating what you're experiencing. Pay attention to how you're speaking to yourself and others, what you're doing, what your attitude is, who you're spending your time with, and if you react or respond. If what you're doing and who you're being is not nourishing or uplifting, and if who you're spending time with is not helpful, encouraging, and uplifting, then it's time to tweak and adjust.

Nothing changed for the better until I ...

1. Took responsibility for what was showing up in my life. **Everything** showing up, I was responsible for.
2. Started to be aware of what I was doing, how I was speaking, who I was being, and the energy I was giving out.
3. Started to make uplifting, helpful, and nourishing choices (**especially in my attitude**) to bring about more positive, uplifting, and nourishing results.
4. Chose to have faith, appreciation, and trust in the process of life, instead of fear, anger, doubt, guilt, and regret. Fear, doubt, guilt, anger, and regret did not bring me great results. As a matter of fact, it was a miserable place to live and not a good use of my energy. Faith,

trust, and appreciation **changed my life** and will change yours! **No good will come from giving your world negative feelings and emotions. No good will come from giving yourself negative feelings and emotions.** When you really "get" this, it will change your world. You will start to move into your world from your spirit with the energy of *love* and all its related emotions, not from ego with the energy of *fear* and all its related emotions.

It's not very fun getting kicked around by life. It's even less fun when you're making choices that aren't helping you move in a positive direction. Then it seems like life is really out to get you, but it's really *you* that's getting in your own way. How do we get in our own way? With a victim mentality.

We've all been there. We blame everyone and everything for our hard time. However, when you stop the blaming and take a look at yourself, when you walk through the tough times, when you dig in deep and figure your shit out, when you look back and "get" the lesson life is teaching you and grow stronger from it, it's these times that you really learn to appreciate because it makes you stronger for yourself and others. You also learn a lot about yourself, what choices you made, the outcome of those choices, and how you would choose differently from this point on. Life is all about choosing, experiencing, learning, and growing. There is *always* a result to every choice you make. And that result doesn't just affect you, but the world around you. When you start owning your choices, you start really enjoying your life because you need to be present in the moment to choose, and when you're present in the moment, you find you're able to appreciate and experience what's happening that much more.

I'm going to share with you one of my major "Oh crap, what did I do?" experiences and one of my "Are you kidding me?" experiences. My intention is to inspire and motivate you to pay attention to your choices and to be aware of the consequences of those choices.

It's definitely easier to "see" and understand choice/consequence or the spiritual law of cause and effect when you look at what other people are experiencing or have experienced because of the choices they've made. We learn from and grow not only from our personal experiences, but also from the experiences of others. I have come to learn that all choices create a result. That's it. We label things as good or bad, or right and wrong. It's still a choice—and a result. But even the "bad" gives us a chance to learn, grow, dig in deep, figure things out, and experience the choices we made. They hopefully make us a stronger, more loving and grateful person.   You experience your choices. That's it. Yes, other people are involved in our world, and yes, outer situations are happening. But we choose how will interpret everything. We choose our perceptions and beliefs. We choose the conversations we have and the words we say. We choose the actions we will take or not take. And we choose our attitudes and how we treat other people and ourselves day in and day out. All of those choices will reap a consequence or result to experience. And on and on life goes.

"Oh crap, what did I do?"

Let me start by saying I was blessed to experience a very loving, supportive, and happy childhood. My parents had a loving marriage and always showed respect to each other. I am one of five siblings, and we all got along although we were very different in our personalities. Mom stayed home and took care of us and the house. Dad worked hard in his own business, was successful, and loved spending time with us, especially on Sundays. Sundays were sacred. Our parents were supportive, encouraging, and tough when they needed to be.

As a teenager, I loved all forms of movement and exercise, especially dance. I joined the school dance company and loved practicing, performing, and being part of such a disciplined group. I found my love becoming an obsession. We had weigh-ins every week, and I remember being so proud of myself for easily losing weight (even though I didn't need to) and getting praise and attention because of it.   Well … I started being very calculated with my food intake. I was eating healthy, but eating very little. You can probably guess the consequence that under-nourishing myself led to. My body just said enough. I literally couldn't get out of bed one morning without passing out. My parents were beside themselves, and I actually saw my dad cry. My body not being able to move (which I loved to do) and my parents getting emotional were enough motivation for me to make a change. I couldn't eat more, because I developed a habit of eating such small, calculated quantities. So, I decided to make nourishing shakes. This worked for me. I eventually gained enough weight to look normal and not undernourished, and I eventually started to eat more and develop a healthier relationship with myself and food.

I vowed I would never, ever mistreat my body like that again. I said sorry to God for mistreating my body. Our body is the outer shell that houses our spirit. Whatever your religion or spiritual journey is, our body is a blessing … no matter what it looks like, no matter what state of health it's in. It's a blessing, and it's your responsibility to take care of it. Own that responsibility by owning your choices. To live in a healthy, energized, and vibrant body makes life enjoyable, fun, and exciting. Understand, under-nourishing your body by not eating enough, or by eating too much processed junk food, fast food, or packaged food will cause illness to the body. It's not a matter of if; it's a matter of when.

What growth did I experience?

We all have a relationship with food, and you have to decide whether yours is nourishing and healthy, or not. If not, you have to decide to make some changes one step at a time. It can be done; I did it. I embraced the fact that my body is the temple that houses my true self, my spirit. And not taking care of my body leads to sickness and pain—both physical and emotional pain. Our emotions are very strong, and when you allow those emotions to dictate what to eat, how much to eat, or anything having to do with food, you find yourself in an unhealthy relationship with food. Food is meant to be enjoyed and nourishing for the body, not to fill a void in your life.

Have you been mistreating your body by your food choices? How is your relationship with food?

Is your relationship with food healthy and nourishing? What can you do now to take steps toward a healthier relationship? What is your inner voice telling you?

Every day is a new opportunity to commit yourself to healthy, nourishing, and uplifting choices not only in food, but in what you say, what you do, how you think, and the attitudes you bring to each moment. It's all connected, and each choice matters. The food you eat affects your attitude, and your attitude affects the food you eat. Every choice matters.

"Are you f——— kidding me?"

My dad died of a heart attack when I was twenty-one years old. He was fifty-one. This literally knocked me to my knees, more times than I can count. It was something I just couldn't understand. He was a healthy, vibrant, loving-life kind of man. My family's rock. We were all very, very close to him. I just couldn't understand how and why this happened. He was young, took care of himself, and had a successful business and loving family. I literally found myself looking up at the sky, and saying, "What the f———?"

I was angry. I was mad at God for taking him away from us, angry at the world for carrying on like nothing happened, and angry at the sun for rising the next morning after his funeral. You name it, I was mad. I was in pain and didn't know how to handle it. I hurt everyone close to me and made some major life choices in anger and pain. When the dust settled, after about two years of living in anger and pain, I woke up one morning with no job, no friends, no family, no husband, and no money. My choices had brought me to rock bottom.

I remember as clearly as if it were yesterday, hitting my knees one night and sobbing. I just kept saying, "Please God, help me. I made a mess." I fell asleep crying and praying, and I woke up the next morning to a peace I will never ever forget. It was an inner peace and a *knowing* that everything was going to be okay. I remember feeling very, very grateful for this knowing. This wasn't just a belief; this was a knowing. I had no doubt in my mind that God was with me and that I didn't need to be afraid, even though my circumstances were such a mess. I chose to forgive myself since I really felt that God forgave me. The first thing I did was ask for forgiveness from my family, my ex-husband, and my boss. My family embraced me, my ex-husband forgave me, and my boss took me back as a personal trainer. I decided to live in gratitude for this second chance, to give thanks to God each and every day, not only for the knowing of peace within me, but for walking with me each day. I knew and still know that no matter what, I will always be okay and provided for. I feel a deep sense of appreciation even to this day for my family, my health, God getting me back on track, for my work, for every single thing in my life.   Living from a place of peace and gratitude changed my life. My personal training business took off, I met my best friend who is now my husband, I remain close with my family, and I having loving and supportive people around me. I didn't visualize. I didn't set goals. I just prayed, gave thanks, and trusted. Prayed, gave thanks, and trusted. I took action from this place of appreciation and trust.

Pray/meditate, give thanks, and trust in the unfolding of life.

I still do the same practice now. *Pray/meditate, give thanks, and trust in the unfolding of life.*

How did I grow from this? Oh my, where do I start?

I learned to never, ever take anyone or anything for granted. Love your life and everyone in it because it can change in an instant. I didn't have any control over my dad passing. I didn't cause it, and I didn't bring this to pass. However, the way I reacted caused a lot of pain and destruction. If I would have found healthier ways to express and release my pain, the outcome would have been very different. I have learned to practice faith and trust that there is a bigger picture unfolding in the scheme of life. The attitude of appreciation I practiced every day changed my life.

I learned that although anger and other negative emotions are a normal part of life, giving your world these emotions—allowing yourself to linger there and moving from that place of negativity—is destructive. No good can come from it. There are healthier ways to release and let go of these emotions, which we will talk about, but acting and choosing from a place of anger, resentment, and other negativity will bring about negative consequences. Get calm and peaceful first. Then make your choices and decisions. Try to never act and make decisions from a place of negativity. It just brings you pain and heartache, and it brings the world around you pain and heartache.

I learned to trust that everything will be okay. No matter what's going on, trust that God has your back and that everything is unfolding as it should. Even when you don't understand. Pray, give thanks, and trust. Meditate, love, and trust. Trust in the process and journey called life. We are spiritual beings, and we have come here to love, enjoy, experience, learn, and grow. Obstacles, tragedies, accidents, and disease will be a part of everyone's life. As the Bible tells us, there is a time to experience everything under the sun. "There is a time for everything, and a season for every activity under heaven. A time to be born and a time to die. A time to plant, and a time to reap. A time to tear down and a time to build up. A time to mourn and a time to dance. A time to weep and a time laugh. A time to be silent and a time to speak. A time to gain and a time to lose." Ecclesiastes 3:1. How will you respond to them? Will it be in trust, appreciation, and love? Or fear, anger, and worry? What will you choose?

Trust the process. You don't need to get knocked to your knees to wake up. Wake up now to the beauty and abundance that you have in your life right now. I'm not implying to deny any troubles you have (whether it's financial, relationship stuff, or whatever); I'm suggesting that you take a look at yourself and start analyzing what you are "giving" and ask yourself if it's nourishing, helpful, and uplifting. If not, make the most nourishing and uplifting choice you can make right now to help shift things to a better place. And then allow your life to unfold. Being worried, angry, blaming, criticizing, and condemning is a miserable place to live. It's not helpful, uplifting, or nourishing. I have a true *knowing* that God is with me, that God is a loving God, and that I can get through anything because he walks right by my side. As long as I stay connected to Spirit, and move from that place, God is with me, and all will always be well no matter what.

I learned that when we're experiencing a tragedy or obstacle, it's tempting to feel alone and that God has abandoned us. **Look for the love** no matter what's happening, and that's where God is. Accidents, disease, death of a loved one—no one is immune from experiencing these painful parts of life. But if you look for the love within these tragedies, that's where God is. People coming together and giving my family support, telling us how much my father meant to them—that is love, and there is God. In the hug and embrace of a family member, in the meals that were provided for us, in the shoulder to cry on, and in the person who was willing to listen to our sorrow. There is God.

There isn't a day that goes by that you don't hear some type of bad news either from another person, or from the news, or whatever. But wherever there is "bad" and tragedy, there is a coming together— supporting, caring, tears, love. There is God. Always look and put your attention on the beauty, on the goodness, in the kindness you see and experience, and in the love. There is God in the beauty, the goodness, the love, and the kindness. I now know that God is my rock. And the relationship I had with my father I am forever grateful for. I experienced so much pain when he passed, and that's only because I loved him so much. I am grateful. **Look for the love everywhere**; there is God. God is love. Where there is love, there is God. This keeps you from being overcome with anger, despair, sorrow, etc. *Look for the love in everyone and everything.* What you seek, what you look for, you will find.

WHY CHOOSE TO LIVE
A HEALTHY DAY?

BEFORE WE GO into the five fundamental steps to the *Choose Well to Live Well* lifestyle practice, let's talk a little about why I think it's important to first set an intention to live a healthy day. **We only live one day at a time.** Every decision starts with an intention. An energy focus. Choose to have a healthy day in mind, conversations, actions, and attitude. Why? Our children need us to. They need an example of healthy and happy living, and it starts with us. There's a growing problem among our kids these days, and the statistics are getting worse. I truly believe that if, as adults, we take full responsibility for our health and well-being, it gives the kids in our lives an example to follow.

I am not a proponent of any lose-weight-quickly schemes and programs. I just don't believe there are short cuts to healthy weight loss. I am, however, a huge proponent of being healthy. If the lose-weight-quickly schemes worked, we wouldn't be in the health crisis we're experiencing. The weight-loss industry is a multibillion-dollar industry, and it's not making us any healthier. Trying the newest and latest fad diet is not the healthiest choice. It may even cause more harm than good. I believe that if our society made an attitude adjustment from "weight loss" to choosing to "be healthy," we would shift to having a healthier country. You would be patient with your body instead of bringing frustration and impatience into your moment because changes are not happening fast enough.

Just make the decision to choose healthy now, today.

The Scary CDC (Center for Disease Control) Statistics

We just can't afford to have an obese, ill population anymore. It's time to live one day at a time, making the healthier choices possible.

To say that obesity is serious, common, and costly is an understatement. In 2009–2010, more than one-third of the US adults were obese. That's 35.7 percent!

The health consequences of obesity are cardiovascular disease, high blood pressure, high levels of triglycerides (fat) in the blood and around major organs, stroke, high cholesterol, Type 2 diabetes, cancer, sleep disorders, liver and gallbladder disease, osteoarthritis, and gynecological problems.

As body weight increases, the risk of disease increases. Not only that, but instead of taking our health and well-being into our own hands and under our control, we go to prescriptive drugs, and the interaction of five or more prescriptions can be deadly because of the combination. Meanwhile, if you just clean up your eating, get moving, and start managing your state of mind and emotions, your body will heal itself to a healthier state—**given the chance.**

Our children need us to be healthy examples. Obesity now affects 17 percent of all children and adolescents. It's actually tripled from just a generation ago. Children are now getting diagnosed with heart disease, diabetes, and breathing problems as teenagers! It's crazy. There needs to be a shift, and it needs to start with us as adults. When you get healthier in mind and body, everyone around you benefits.

I also feel we are too illness conscious. Our society has a tendency to focus on the symptoms and treat those symptoms with drugs—without looking at the possible causes so you won't experience the illness again. We have so many specialists that treat specific parts of our body, but our body works as a whole. We need to start shifting our consciousness and attention away from illness and disease and toward wellness and health. Watch any TV program, and you're bombarded with drug commercials asking you to ask your doctor about the drug if you're experiencing a list of symptoms. Meanwhile, the drugs just treat the symptoms without getting to the *cause* of what you're experiencing—which is most likely your lifestyle.

Wellness consciousness means putting all your attention on wellness. It's about taking a look at the choices you're making as a result of your lifestyle, which is causing the symptoms. Dehydration, lack of sleep, not enough movement, unhealthy eating habits, and constant feelings of worry and stress cause all sorts of physical symptoms. The body can heal itself with effort, patience, and awareness. Good health and well-being is our natural state. Our body wants to be healthy and thrive. It knows how to fight illness and disease when it has too. That's what our immune system is for. But let's start being helpful to our immune system by choosing to practice daily the five fundamentals to support our natural state of health and wellness.

Let's now talk about how we create our world and how we experience the results of our choices.

> *Setting an example is not the main means of*
> *influencing others, it is the only means.*
> **—Albert Einstein**

Choice and Consequence

What are we choosing? What are the results of those choices?

Make a choice. Experience the consequence and result of that choice. All choices will reap a consequence/result. That result is what you will experience. From that experience, you make more choices. That is a basic explanation of the spiritual law of cause and effect. All religions and spiritual practices teach this basic law in one way or another. According to Galatians 5:7, "Man reaps what he sows."

Positive, uplifting, nourishing, and helpful choices reap you positive, nourishing, and uplifting consequences and results. You will feel positive emotions and feelings and attract more positive experiences to you.

Negative, toxic, unhealthy choices reap you negative, toxic, and unhealthy consequences. You will feel negative emotions and feelings and attract more negativity to you.

It is as simple as that. **You get and experience what you give.** Cause someone deliberate hurt and pain, and you will experience the same. Show love, compassion, and kindness, and you will experience the same.

We are creating our own personal world and experiences at the same time everyone else is creating their world, so there is a *bigger picture* happening, and that's where the trust comes in. We are co-creating with everyone around us. We are all connected. When something happens, and you don't get it, **just trust.** (Which is what I should have done when my father died.) Just trust that there's a bigger plan, and everything that happens is meant to happen. **There are no accidents.** We are all in this world together, and we are all connected. What may seem like a negative situation may just be the best thing that has ever happened to you. **Ride it out with the best attitude and energy you can.** Breathe, pray, meditate, take action, hang on, and trust. We are all here to experience life.

Meditate, pray, give thanks and love, and trust. Know that everything unfolds for the good of the whole. There is always good that comes from something that is seemingly bad. You can find *love* everywhere. There is always a blessing in each and every situation, but sometimes you have to look for it to find it. You will always find what you are looking for. Look for the love in a situation, and you will find it. Look for something to complain about and be angry about, and you will find it. Whatever you are looking for, you will find. Look for the good, and you will find it. Where is your attention? What are you looking for?

You always have a choice.

> *For every minute you are angry, you*
> *lose sixty seconds of happiness.*
> —*Ralph Waldo Emerson*

Every thought, word, action, and attitude you choose to give is a "cause" that creates the "effect" or physical experience and circumstance. When you choose to move from your spirit, and you give thoughts, words, actions, and attitudes of love, joy, peace, calmness, hope, trust, optimism, and other positive feelings, it results in good health in your physical body, a boosted immune system, and experiences that are happy, joyful, and peaceful.

When you choose to move from your ego, and you give thoughts, words, actions, and attitudes characterized by a victim mentality, lack-consciousness, anger, frustration, anxiety, worry, and other negative emotions, it results in a depressed immune system, it sets up an environment in your body for disease and un-wellness, and it creates more negative situations to experience.

Anger, worry, and stress produce more anger, worry, and stress to experience. It is not helpful to any situation or circumstance. It is toxic energy that affects not only your body and mind, but everyone around you.

You have to change a "cause" in order to change the "effect." Always be aware and pay attention to your attitude—what you are thinking, how you feel, what you say, and what you do. These are all "causes" that determine what you experience and how life unfolds. Ask yourself if you're giving yourself and your world the most helpful and uplifting "causes" that you can in each moment.

Every human being is the author of
his own health or dis-ease.
—Buddha

To get up each morning with the resolve to be
happy is to set our own conditions to the events of
each day. To do this is to condition circumstances
instead of being conditioned by them.
—Ralph Waldo Emerson

THE FIVE FUNDAMENTALS TO CREATE A FIT, STRONG, HEALTHY BODY AND STATE OF MIND

1. Change what you can control. What you think, say, do, and the attitude you bring—these are all under your control and can be changed at any time to create a better result.
2. Keep it clean.
3. Move it or lose it.
4. Get quality ZZZ's.
5. Stay hydrated.

EACH FUNDAMENTAL STEP has an effect on the health of our physical body and state of mind. Healthy choices reap healthy results.

When we have **done** our best in each moment, chosen to **be** our best in each moment, and chosen to **think and speak** our best in each moment, then the results will unfold in **peace**.

I have always loved the Serenity Prayer. "God grant me the serenity to accept the things I cannot change, courage to change the things I can, and the wisdom to know the difference." There is such beauty and goodness in this prayer. Digging in deep and choosing to trust and accept all things you have no control over, and digging in deep for the courage and strength to make the changes you can by controlling what you can. Accept what you must, and change what you need to change—whether it's how you think, what you believe, what you say and do, or the attitude you bring to each aspect of life. This prayer and meditation puts us in charge of our health, our happiness, and the choices we make in our life.

Can it be this simple? Yes, but let me ask you: are *you* practicing these steps on a daily basis? If more people were practicing these basic steps, we wouldn't be in the health care crisis we are experiencing right now and we would have a lot of happy, healthy people experiencing life! Just focusing on one of these steps on a consistent basis will improve your health and well-being. I stand by this 100 percent and am dedicated to living these five steps day in and day out. I am also dedicated to helping my clients live these steps day in and day out. Will you choose to live these five steps each day?

> *Every day is a new opportunity to move*
> *yourself in the right direction.*
> *Though no one can go back and make a brand-new start,*
> *anyone can start from now and make a brand-new ending.*
> **—Anonymous**

Understand that all of your choices will affect how you feel, and how you feel affects your choices. The five choose-well fundamentals are interconnected. Each step affects the other steps either positively or negatively, depending on the quality of your choices.

In other words, if you work late on the computer and don't shut down from all input and stimulation before bed, you won't sleep well. It can be caused by either too much input, worrying thoughts running through your mind, or anxiety about all you need to accomplish the next day. If you don't sleep well, you are making it tougher on yourself to keep a positive, optimistic outlook because you don't feel well. If you don't sleep well, you may not make the best food choices. If you don't sleep well, you won't have the energy to exercise. The reverse is also true. If you don't exercise consistently, you may not sleep well because you didn't release tension and stress from your body, and you'll make it a bit more difficult to manage your state of mind because your body doesn't feel well because of lack of exercise and too much pent-up stress held in it. Your body needs to move in order to get proper rest. Your body needs to move to release emotional stress. Your body needs to move in order to be strong and fit.

If you don't exercise because you think you have no time, your body will be in pain or get sick, and you won't feel well. If you don't feel well, it's hard to be patient and calm. If you don't drink enough water or drink too much coffee, you may experience headaches, cramps, constipation, and exhaustion. When you experience these things, you may reach for medication, which makes things worse for your body because of the side effects of the meds and because the real cause of your symptoms is dehydration.

If you eat like crap, you feel like crap. And when you feel like crap, you're just making it tougher to bring a good attitude to all moments of your life. If you eat like crap, you won't sleep well or have the proper energy for a good workout.

If you're bored, lonely, or upset, you may reach for food to comfort you. If you reach for food to comfort you, you will feel guilty afterwards. Feeling guilty is not a helpful emotion for you or for your body, and you will reach for more food, alcohol, or drugs to numb yourself so that you won't feel what you feel and face what needs to be faced. I think you get the point. These are just a few examples to show how these steps are tied to one another. So, it's really important to pay attention to your choices within each of the five steps, and the results of those choices, so you can tweak and start choosing better. Work with all five of these steps together.

Again, food choices affect the way you feel. Exercise affects the way you feel. Hydration affects the way you feel. Quality sleep affects the way you feel.

The thoughts you think affect the way you feel. The conversations you have affect the way you feel. Your attitude and mood affect the way you feel. Your behavior and actions affect the way you feel. These are all "causes" that determines your "effect" or outcome.

The way you feel determines how your life unfolds … **and all five choose-well steps affect the way you feel!**

A change in how you feel brings a change in the events and circumstances you experience.

Fundamental One: Change and Control What You Can. What Can We Change and Control?

YOUR THOUGHTS AND the beliefs you have about yourself, your body, your relationships, your work, your health, and the world can be changed in an instant, and therefore your life can be changed in an instant. Your thoughts are energy, and they begin the creation process of everything you experience. Start thinking in a more uplifting, helpful, and encouraging way that's in line with what you want to accomplish. These thoughts create an uplifting, encouraging, good feeling.

Our thoughts create our experiences. Our thoughts affect every cell in our body. Healthy thoughts = healthy cells = healthy and fit body and state of mind. Unhealthy, worried, negative thoughts = unhealthy cells = disease, illness, pain in the body, and an anxious state of mind.

What we think, we become.
—Buddha

One thought leads to heaven; one thought leads to hell.
—Buddha
*Only when we change our thoughts about a
situation will our behavior and results change.*
—Albert Einstein

As a man thinketh within himself, so is he.
—Proverbs 23:7

The images and pictures you play in your mind about yourself, your body, your relationships, your work, your finances, your health, and the world are under your control. We think in mental pictures. Plant uplifting and nourishing images in your mind every day for how you want your relationships, the health of your physical body, and the health of your finances and work to be. Feel all the positive emotions in your physical body as if what you intend is already a reality for you. Feel the joy, contentment, excitement, energy, and enthusiasm. Take time every day with this practice of imaging and feeling, and make sure they are supportive, helpful, and in line with your intentions, desires, and goals.

Always practice imagining a good outcome to whatever situation comes your way. You are going to contemplate something, so you might as well make it the most uplifting, helpful, and nourishing contemplation you can!

Be vigilant; guard your mind against negative thoughts.
—Buddha

The words you speak to others and what you say to yourself are your responsibility and in your control. If you want to know what you've been thinking, start paying attention to what you're saying. Make a commitment to yourself right now to **stop blaming, complaining, condemning, and criticizing yourself and others— and to start appreciating**. Speak positively and optimistically. This one practice changed my life. Only speak what is helpful, uplifting, and nourishing. That's it. Only have conversations that are helpful, uplifting, and nourishing. Watch your words. How you speak is how you think. Speak only goodness.

Words have the power to both destroy and heal.
When words are both true and kind,
they can change our world.
—Buddha

Do not let any unwholesome talk come out of your mouths,
but only what is helpful for building others up according to
their needs, that it may benefit those who listen.
—**Ephesians 4:29**

The actions you choose to take or not to take are your responsibility and under your control. We are such a "do" society that I think we sometimes neglect the attitude we're giving as we're doing! Not paying attention to what you're giving is the number-one reason we get in our own way of achieving any goal or dream. That and not taking any action at all! You can't just work like crazy without checking in with yourself and paying attention to the energy you're giving behind that action. If you're working hard at a goal and seeing no results, check in with your attitude. You may be bringing an attitude of frustration, anger, or worry and getting in your own way with this attitude. Make a shift to a more encouraging, uplifting, and nourishing attitude. Action is important. But your intended state of being is just as important. Check in with yourself. Take care not to give any situation or circumstance negative energy. It just creates more negativity for you to experience.

I can do all things through him who strengthens me.
—**Philippians 4:13**

Everything is based on the mind, is led by the mind,
is fashioned by mind. If you speak and act with a
polluted mind, suffering will follow you, as the wheels
of the oxcart follow the ox. Everything is based on
the mind, is led by the mind, is fashioned by mind.
If you speak and act with a pure mind, happiness
will follow you, as a shadow clings to a form.
—**Buddha**

The attitude you bring to each and every day, to each and every situation, and to each and every moment is a choice you make. Are you cultivating an optimistic, appreciative attitude? Or are you bringing a victim attitude? What are you choosing? Are you getting in your own way with a negative attitude? Again, this is the energy you're giving. When you give positive, kind, loving energy, you receive back from the world kind, loving, and positive results. **The solution to any problem, unwanted situation, or circumstance is always found in a change of attitude and focus.** A change in attitude and focus brings about a change in feeling. A change in feeling brings about a change in experience.

If we could see the miracle of a single flower
clearly, our whole life would change.
—Buddha

Live a life of love.
—Ephesians 5:2

In a nutshell: Control and manage how you think, how you speak, your behavior and actions, and your attitude. These are *yours* to choose and control—not anyone else's. When you take responsibility for these choices, you take responsibility for your life.

VICTIM OR CREATOR

The source of all of our problems arises
from our mental afflictions.
—Dalia Lama

Holding on to anger is like grasping a hot
coal with the intent of throwing it at someone
else, yet you are the one getting burned.
—Buddha

*We can let circumstances rule us, or we can take
charge and rule our lives from within.*
—Earl Nightingale

Pay attention and wake up to how you are showing up in your life. This is the beginning of being a creator in your world. Pay attention to the people you spend your time with and how you speak. How you are speaking is how you are thinking.

How do you know if you are being a victim in life? If you find yourself blaming, complaining, criticizing, condemning, gossiping, comparing, judging , worrying, angry, or resentful at yourself, other people, or the whatever the moment is bringing you, you are pretty much hanging out in a victim mentality, and it's a miserable place to be. Blaming gives your power away to the person or circumstance you are blaming. Blame, judgment, and criticism create victims. If you don't take back your power to choose a healthier, uplifting, and nourishing state of being and attitude, and you linger in negative states, you will bring more situations and circumstances in your life to keep you stuck in this victim mentality, and your physical body will get sick. You need to deliberately choose not to be a victim of your circumstances and other people. You need to choose not to be a victim of other people's "stuff" that they have to figure out. You can be encouraging and helpful, but choose not to be an enabler of their mentality. Practice being someone different. Practice choosing the attitude and energy you want to give in every moment, instead of blaming your surroundings for your unease and frustration. We are so quick to blame someone else for how we feel. You lose all your power when you blame. It is so easy be a victim. What is not so easy is accepting that we are responsible for our thoughts, behaviors, and attitudes that are causing our feelings.

People who give their world a victim mentality also tend to not take any action to make their situation or experience better. They tend to be problem-oriented, focused on their problems, what they're lacking, and what's not going right for them. They also tend to look back and blame and complain about the past, thereby infecting their moment and their future. They tend to relive unwanted things and circumstances over and over again.

Creators cultivate optimism and put positive action behind their decisions. They do so expecting a good outcome, trusting that all will work out well, and acknowledging the good in their life right here and right now. Creators are solution-oriented. They watch what they say, how they think, and manage their attitude. Creators make sure their attitudes, conversations, and actions are helpful, uplifting, and encouraging. They keep clear of negativity and victims. Creators discipline themselves to respond instead of react. Creators never give up on themselves or their goals. Creators are aware of where their time, energy, and attention are going. Creators make sure most of their time is spent with people who uplift and encourage them, and not with those who drain them of their energy. Creators choose how they will perceive a situation. Creators choose what attitude they will give their world. Creators choose to respond instead of react to situations and circumstances. Being happy and healthy is a choice that creators deliberately choose.

Be in charge of your thoughts. Be in charge of how you speak. Be in charge of your behavior, and be in charge of the attitude you give. No matter what, no blaming, criticizing, or condemning.

You always have the choice to create your day or to be a victim of your circumstances and other people. You can choose to remain in a state of peace and calmness no matter what's going on around you. What others do, say, and think are reflections of their own inner state. Choose not to be a victim of others' actions and words. That is their responsibility, and it is up to them to experience their choices. Figure out your own, work through your own, and own your power to choose. Allow them to experience their own choices. Give them your prayers, good thoughts, and send them love. Even when you think they don't deserve it. Why? Because *you* deserve it. It frees you from being a victim of others. Don't give your power away.

Excuses and justifications keep you stuck in a victim mentality. And remember, the law of choice/consequence is always at work. Tend to your own choices, and allow others to tend to theirs. Just keep a picture in mind of you being the center of your own personal world. You are the center of your relationships, of your work/career, and your physical body. What you choose to be, do, and say affects everything. Will you be a victim of your world, or a creator of your world?

Practice

Refuse to complain, judge, criticize, or condemn yourself, others, and the present moment. **Just stop**. When you catch yourself, **take a timeout**. Just take a breath, regroup, and stop speaking. Just stop. Refuse to entertain and contemplate any negative, destructive, or fearful idea or thought. Rise above anything or anyone that attempts to anger you, worry you, or make you fearful. Choose faith, trust, and calmness over fear, doubt, worry, and anger. **It is a choice.**

Stop the complaining and **start giving** positive, nurturing energy to your world. Love, peace, appreciation, kindness, optimism, and calmness are beautiful states of being and attitudes that will change your life. You can develop your own practice of nurturing attitudes. Please keep in mind that it takes practice and a never-give-up attitude to break out of a victim mentality, especially if you developed a habit of showing up in your world this way. You need to consciously and deliberately practice a different attitude until it becomes a natural way of being for you. Be patient.

Worry = Fear

Stress = Fear

What are we afraid of? Not being enough, not having enough, not enough time to get everything done, failing, succeeding, eating, loving, caring, being happy. Whatever it is, you can choose to have faith and trust. Understand that when you have this energy of worry, fear, and stress, it just attracts more circumstances to be worried, fearful, and stressed out about. Not only that, but it is toxic to every cell of our body, which sets us up for illness, pain, and disease. How many times have you experienced digestive issues, headaches, or back/neck pain after feeling emotionally stressed about something? It's not a coincidence. **Practice another attitude and energy.**

Worry and stress are not helpful for anyone or any situation. If you're concerned about a loved one or about a situation you're experiencing, send out love to that situation. Shift to a more helpful energy, whatever feels right for you. Even if it's repeating a mantra: "This too shall pass," or "All is well in my life," or "I choose to live in faith, trust, and appreciation over fear, doubt, and worry." If sending love is a stretch for you right now, at the very least, be hopeful. Contemplate a good outcome. Keep telling yourself to live one day at a time. Do and be your best, and allow God to handle the rest.

It's not that hard to understand, and it's not that hard to figure out what to tweak and change. What is not so easy is to make a daily commitment to change what you can, and to allow things to unfold as they should. What is not so easy is dropping the excuses and justifications as to why you're moving in your world as a victim. What is not so easy is getting honest with yourself and finally making the decision to own your part in creating the circumstances you're experiencing. What is not so easy is changing a victim habit and creating a new, healthier one. What is not so easy is staying centered in your chosen state of being while others around you are being victims in life. Simple, not always easy. It takes a deep intention and desire to want to change. Practice the change daily. And do not give up until you have created a healthier habit, and your life begins to shift.

Your thoughts, mental pictures, words, actions, and attitudes all create feelings inside of you. And the way you feel creates the experiences you live. When you change the way you feel, you change your world. When you start making conscious choices that deliberately nourish and uplift you and those around you, you feel good. It's a beautiful thing going through life feeling good and happy.

There's only one way anger *may* be helpful for you. It's when it motivates you to make positive changes in your life. When you finally become sick and tired of your physical body being sick, tired, or overweight, and you do something about it. When you stand up for yourself and have had enough of someone being unkind, and you remove yourself from the situation and say, "Enough, I am not going to be treated this way anymore." When you are tired of worrying about your finances and become proactive and do something about it. But as soon as you make that decision, motivated by anger, shift out of that state to a more "uplifted" one to help yourself along the journey toward good health and well-being.

Think about this: Have anger, blaming, condemning, or criticizing ever produced peaceful results? Have anger, blaming, condemning, or criticizing ever produced happiness? Have anger, blaming, condemning, or criticizing ever produced a healthy body? All thinking, speaking, behaviors, and attitude are the result of **choice**. When we accept responsibility for our every thought, behavior, attitude, and the way we speak, we **empower** ourselves.

> *Feeling sorry for yourself and for your present*
> *condition is not only a waste of energy,*
> *but the worst habit you could possibly have.*
> **—Dale Carnegie**

There is power in choosing. Own it. Be conscious. Pay attention.

CHOOSE-WELL QUESTIONS

When you start asking yourself questions, you automatically become present to your life, you bring awareness to what is going on, and you can start changing what can be changed and is in your control. When you start asking questions, you become more aware of the choices you're making and whether you want to experience the result of those choices.

What energy am I choosing to give (to myself, my relationships, my physical body, and my work through my thoughts, images, words, actions, and attitudes)?

Is this choice nourishing, uplifting, and helpful? Or negative, toxic, and destructive to all aspects of my life?

You are either choosing to give good thoughts, images, words, attitudes, and actions to all aspects of your life *or not*. Remember, there is always a result for each and every choice you make. And you have to start asking yourself if you want to experience the result of your choice. Nourishing and uplifting choices reap you positive results.

I love the words *nourishing* and *uplifting*. The dictionary defines them as follows:

Nourish—"to cherish, strengthen, build up and promote. To supply with what is necessary for life, health and growth."

Uplift—"to raise, elevate, inspire, offering encouragement, providing hope. The process or work of improving."

I love the energy behind the words. It is a positive and loving choice. In everything you are about to do, say, think, and be, ask yourself these questions. It will keep you in an uplifted and positive state of being. When you practice living one moment at a time and choose in each moment that which is uplifting and nourishing for you and your life, you will find yourself enjoying and loving your life.

When you make nourishing and uplifting choices, not only do you benefit, but the world benefits. We are all connected. And what you choose has a ripple effect that is endless. One kind word, one kind act, can reach so many people in one day. It is not only a self-care choice, but I believe it's a world-care choice. Nourishing thoughts, words, actions, and attitudes strengthen you, build you up, and keep you in a state of feeling good. It really means **love**.

When you nourish yourself, you **give** nourishing thoughts, words, actions, and attitudes that are kind, loving, supportive, helpful, and optimistic to yourself, your goals, and your dreams.

When you nourish and uplift your relationships, you **give** kind, loving, supportive, helpful, and optimistic thoughts, words, actions, and attitudes.

When you nourish your body, you choose clean whole foods to eat, plenty of fresh water to drink, and you choose to move and sweat every day to get rid of the toxins that accumulate in your body.

You speak words that are helpful, nourishing, and uplifting to build healthy cells in the body.

When you nourish and uplift your work, career, and finances, you **give** confident, positive, optimistic, excited thoughts, words, actions, and attitudes toward your goals, bills, and finances.

The CDC (Center for Disease Control) now says that 99 percent of all disease and illnesses is caused by stress. A simple definition of stress is seeing it as an emotional reaction to what's going on in your life. Stress is self-created because it's your choice and your reaction that are causing the stress response. It makes sense to learn and practice how to manage your emotions and feelings in order to create a fit, healthy, and strong mind and body.   It also has been said that 75 percent of overeating may be linked to emotional eating. Again, it just makes sense to manage your emotions and state of mind!

Spirit—blessings consciousness and love—results in a healthy body and mind.

Peace, joy, appreciation, faith, enthusiasm, passion, kindness, positive expectation, happiness, and all other positive emotions are really expressions of **love**. So too are hope, calmness, optimism, contemplating a good outcome, trusting that all will work out for your best interests, an attitude that things will improve, and knowing that "this too shall pass."

Ego—lack-consciousness, fear, and victim-consciousness— results in a diseased and ill body and mind.

Disappointment, feeling overwhelmed, doubt, frustration, criticizing, condemning, blaming, unkindness, worry, anger, revenge, jealousy, hatred, guilt, despair, depression, and any other negative emotion are really expressions of **fear**.

What am I choosing to give? Is this choice nourishing, helpful, and uplifting? If you find yourself feeling and giving energy in lack-consciousness, make a daily effort and practice "uplifting" your thoughts, attitudes, perceptions, and actions to hope, calmness, and optimism.

How is your attitude? How do you speak? How do you think? How do you behave? Are they helpful and nourishing for your goals and dreams? Who are you spending your time with? Are they uplifting, encouraging, and helpful to you? Do you have some cleaning up to do? Just start now, from where you are with what's going on. Right now, start making helpful, nourishing, and uplifting choices. If you find yourself lingering and hanging out in fear/stress emotions, strive each day to reach for hopefulness.

When we respond negatively to any experience, situation, or circumstance, we have moved away from our spirit and allowed the ego to take charge. Our calmness, inner peace, and at-ease state have disappeared. Be in charge of your thinking, be in charge of your feelings, be in charge of your responses, and make an effort to come from your spirit. Only goodness will result from giving your world your spirit. It is **your daily choice** to give your world your spirit or your ego.

When you are choosing blessings-consciousness instead of the lower energies of lack-consciousness, you are not looking for things to be offended by, and you are not judging or criticizing or labeling others. You are in a state of calmness and grace in which you know you are connected to your spirit, your higher power, God, and you are free from the negative effects of anyone or anything that tries to disrupt your chosen state of being.

If you are feeling anger toward something or someone, and sending them love and forgiveness is a stretch for you **right now**, at the very least, you can **stop** talking about them with anger and hatred. You can put your attention on something that makes you happy and calm.

If you are concerned and worried about someone going through a tough time, they don't need your worried energy. The most helpful, nourishing, and uplifting thing you can do for them is see them as making it through their hard time and see them becoming stronger. Send them prayers and good energy. Send them loving thoughts.

If your physical body needs weight loss, engage in an exercise program and eating program **along with an optimistic attitude that your body will change to a healthy, fit state from your effort**.

How much sense does it make to work out, eat well, and complain that results are not coming fast enough, or to claim that "Nothing is working. I try and just can't drop the weight."? How helpful do you think these thoughts and words are to your goals? Expect your body to lose weight; expect your body to get healthy from the positive changes you are making. Support your efforts with helpful, uplifting, and nourishing thoughts, conversations, and attitudes.

If you are going through a tough financial situation or tough work situation, refuse to give any worry energy, and be hopeful that everything will turn out for your best interest, and know that this too shall pass. Be solution-oriented. Just do and be your best and let God and the universe handle the rest. Focus on the goodness. Put your best effort forward and take action with the most helpful attitude you can bring. Plan or get professional help for a financial plan, and then work your plan with the most optimistic state of mind you can.

Choose to keep your thoughts, conversations, behavior, and attitudes nourishing, uplifting, and helpful. This keeps your consciousness on wellness, good health, and happiness.

You always have the power of choice.

1,440 MINUTES

These are *your* minutes ... **own them.**

Each morning we are born again. What
we do today is what matters most.
—Buddha

Each day is a new opportunity for a new beginning. We are blessed with a clean slate. A new set of 1,440 minutes to choose how we will live, what we will do, what energy we will choose to bring each moment, what we will say, and how we will invest our time. Practice living in the present moment and being here right now. Practice using all your senses and putting your whole self into each unfolding moment. Whatever event happened yesterday that pushed your buttons is over, unless you play it over again and again in your mind, which means you are bringing the negative feeling with you. Whatever happened as a child is over, unless you choose to be a victim of your past and allow it have control over you. Your past is gone. Done. If we are haunted by anything in the past, we are choosing to be haunted by it. But how is that helpful to us right now? Nothing from your past can come into your present or your future unless you allow it.

> *The secret of health for both mind and body is not to mourn*
> *the past, worry about the future, or anticipate troubles,*
> *but to live in the present moment wisely and earnestly.*
>
> **—Buddha**

How are you using your 1,440 minutes? Take a look at the answers to your lifestyle questions. Is there anything eating up your precious minutes that you can use for more nourishing and uplifting choices? For example, too much TV? Too much Facebook time? Too much time at work and not enough play? Too much time with people who drain your energy? What changes will you make to start enjoying your 1,440 minutes? How important are the things getting too much of your time, and what are the aspects of your life that are important to you but are not getting enough of your time?

Are you taking time each morning to decide how you are going to feel, no matter what? Are you imagining your day going well? Each morning, are you taking a few minutes to set you intention for how you will show up in your world? Will you be focused, calm, and optimistic? Or will you be scattered, distracted, and cranky? Please don't tell me you can't take a minute of your 1,440 minutes to decide how you will feel today or what kind of energy you will give your world today. If you take the time to set an intention, you won't have to clean up your attitude during the day.

Are you deliberately putting your attention and focus on things that are positive, that you are grateful for, and the things that are going right in your life right now? Or is your focus on what you are lacking and what is not going right? **Where will you choose to put your attention?** Promise yourself that, just for today, you will refuse to think about what is wrong, missing, or lacking in your life. It is emotionally and physically draining. Allow yourself to look at all aspects of your life from a new perspective—a helpful, uplifting, and nourishing perspective.

You can choose to …

1. Actively and intentionally choose the positive energy you will radiate and give your world. Is it love, kindness, patience, gratitude, optimism? Choose what attitude you will give your relationships, your work environment, and the actual work you do. Choose to put your full attention on whatever the task is at the moment. Choose to appreciate and to stop complaining, condemning, criticizing, and whining. When you deliberately approach your day in this way, and refuse to allow yourself to be swayed no matter what, your life will shift dramatically in a most positive way.

2. Choose to be solution-oriented instead of problem-focused. Focusing on your problems brings with it worried and stressful energy and creates more to be worried and stressed about. Look at what is happening, take a breath, and ask yourself, "What can I do now to make this better?" Work your plan, refusing to give it any worried or stressful energy, and work with the most productive and uplifting attitude you can.

3. Keep yourself in check as you live the day. You know when you feel well, at ease, and balanced—and you know when you don't. Ask yourself during the day, "What energy am I choosing to give? And is this the most nourishing, uplifting, and helpful choice I can make?"

4. Respond instead of react. This requires practice, because we are very habit-oriented to react to things that hurt us, or when people aren't doing what we think they should do, or when the present moment is bringing us something we want to resist. We react in negativity. Take a second and choose how you will respond. This keeps you out of the fight-and-flight response that wreaks so much havoc in our body.

5. Live your life fearlessly. What does that mean? Trust, have faith, and refuse to worry.

6. Practice choosing to live in the moment. Do and be your best right here and now. Trust that God has your back. Trust that life has your back. Trust that the universe is on your side. Commit to this daily. Do your part and control/change what you can, and allow God and the universe to do its part. What you give, you receive back. Every choice reaps a result. Pay attention and choose well.

7. Choose to enjoy your life, and choose to bring joy to everyone around you each day.

8. Refuse to allow yourself to linger in negative emotion. Taking responsibility for your feelings means taking responsibility for your life. Feel your feelings, and even when they are negative, don't resist them, **just don't linger**. Allow them to pass by, using the five choose-well practices.

9. Be easy on yourself. Choose to enjoy the journey of creating a happy and healthy life. If you were cranky today, ride it out; tomorrow is a new day to start again. No lingering. Remember that this is a lifestyle practice. Some days will be better than others. Just do the best you can and allow life to unfold. Learn to trust yourself.

10. Look for the love in every moment, in every person, in every situation and circumstance. Where there is love, there is God.

Be where you are; otherwise you miss your life.
—Buddha

Three Reasons to Give Uplifting, Helpful, and Nourishing Attitudes, Words, Thoughts, and Actions During Your 1,440 Minutes

1. Lingering, contemplating , thinking, talking, making decisions, and taking action in negativity or in a victim mentality is toxic to the body, creates disease, is toxic to your relationships and career, and manifests destructive consequences. It has been said that illness and disease are the consequences of your body lingering in a negative state for a long period of time. I am emphasizing **lingering**. We all feel these emotions, and it is important to feel these emotions when they come up and not to stifle them. However, you need to let them pass through you, move on, and *practice* a more nurturing and uplifting attitude (such as gratitude) to put you back into a better, healthier state.

   Lingering and ruminating in negativity means you put yourself in a state of unease and park your attitude and feelings there. Since you're filled with these negative feelings, this is what you're giving your world. Remember, you attract what you give and what you are. There will always be a physical consequence to mental and emotional negativity, whether it's headaches, muscle aches, digestive issues, whatever. Your body will react. Whether it's worry, anger, frustration, resentment, you name it, if it's negative, it's destructive. I have seen relationships destroyed just because people are unkind to each other with their words, and of course they feel justified in their harshness. I have seen serious digestive issues in young, healthy bodies just because of the emotions of worry and regret. I have seen work and finances fall apart for very hard-working people because worry, anger, anxiety, and frustration have taken root, and they move into their world with that negative energy, not thinking clearly. The more you engage in negativity, the more you will experience negativity.

Greek physician Hippocrates taught that negative emotions cause disease and toxins in the body. These emotions, when they linger, influence the immune system negatively. Our body cells are breaking down and building up—either stronger or weaker—as a result of the thoughts we think, the emotions we feel, the foods we eat, and the movement we choose to engage in or not. **These are all under your control.** So, what are you choosing to give? Is it nourishing, uplifting, and helpful?

2. Since **everything** is energy, a victim mentality and negativity will result in you experiencing more of the same. More circumstance, situations, events, and people that are negative will come to you. It is so easy to blame, complain, criticize, and condemn. It is so easy to play victim. It is also a sad way to live and not empowering at all. **No good will result from a negative state of being.** You reap what you sow.

3. It just doesn't feel good going through life as a victim. It has been said that the greatest gift you can give to your loved ones is to be happy. And if you are not, *you* need to change something that is in your control and not wait around for other people or circumstances to change.

Do your part to change what you can, and allow God to take care of the rest.

Live your minutes wisely!

THE FIVE CHOOSE-WELL PRACTICES FOR MANAGING YOUR STATE OF MIND AND EMOTIONS

One: Practice Blessings-Consciousness

I am convinced that the secret to success and happiness in all aspects of your life is to focus **your attention** on your blessings within your relationships, work, finances, and health of your physical body. Put all your attention on what you can appreciate and what makes you smile. Refuse to take your goodness for granted.

Practicing blessings-consciousness puts you in a state and feeling of appreciation and love. You won't be complaining, blaming, or condemning because you will be too busy feeling good about loving and appreciating the goodness in your life. Put your attention and feeling on what makes you smile, on what makes you feel good. This one intention will keep you from taking any goodness in your life for granted.

Consciousness simply means attention. Are you putting your attention on your blessings in life or on what you lack in life?

Here is a suggested morning practice from Norman Vincent Peale: "Start each day by affirming peaceful, contented, and happy attitudes and your days will tend to be pleasant and successful. Such attitudes are active and definite factors in creating satisfactory conditions. Watch your manner of speech then if you wish to develop a peaceful state of mind."

Practice putting your attention and focus on your blessings **each morning**. Make a commitment to start your day with a feeling of appreciation, gratitude, and blessings. Smile as you take 5–10 minutes **in the morning** to mentally reflect and give thanks. After giving thanks, deliberately choose the attitude you will bring to your day. Keep this state of being in your consciousness and attention. Will you be kind? Patient? Loving? Allowing? Calm? Or continue with appreciation? **Choose** and move through your day practicing your chosen state of being.

Contemplate your relationships for a few minutes. Whether it's with yourself, your children, parents, co-workers, or friends, relationships affect your life more than anything else. Being conscious of your blessings within your relationships makes them thrive. Being conscious of what is lacking and not enough is what causes you to blame, complain, criticize, and play victim. To me, having a victim mentality means you're taking your life and everyone for granted, which causes destruction and heartache if not changed. It's all about what you put your attention and focus on. Appreciating your husband is a different energy and attitude than constantly noticing what he lacks, what is missing, and what he is (in your opinion) doing wrong.

Mentally visualize your closest relationships. Contemplate why you feel blessed to have them in your life. Smile and say, "Thank you."

Mentally visualize your day going well for you at work. Imagine that situations at work will turn out well; contemplate a good outcome. Smile and say, "Thank you." Mentally list all the things about work you feel blessed about. What can you appreciate? Even if you are not where you want to be, there is always something you can feel blessed about. Think about it. Smile and say, "Thank you." **Refuse to bring worry energy to any work or financial situation.** Always practice imagining a good outcome. **Refuse to complain, condemn, or criticize.** Stay focused, bring and do your best, and let God handle the rest.

As you take a shower and get yourself ready for your day, give your body a mental blessing. Smile and say, "Thank you for taking care of me throughout the day." The health of our physical body is the most precious thing in our life, and yet it may be the very thing most of us take for granted, until it gives us a wake-up call. Without good health, we have nothing. You need to start acknowledging and giving thanks to the health of your body, right now. Think about it. Be thankful for your physical senses that allow you to experience your world. The very act of breathing, digesting, and blood circulation happen with us even thinking about them. What a miracle. What a gift! When was the last time you said "thank you" and really appreciated your body? You can walk, feel, and breathe. Smile, put one hand on your heart, one hand on your belly, take a deep breath, and say, "Thank you!" Feeling blessed for what your body does for you keeps you in wellness-consciousness. **Refuse to take your body for granted, or you may lose the health of it.**

Choose to be in a state of blessings-consciousness throughout the day. As you walk through your day and experience all that life has in store for you for this day, notice and give attention to all the things that make you smile, that give you that warm, fuzzy feeling.

In the evening, mentally contemplate all that went well throughout the day. Smile and say, "Thank you." Pick the one thing that made you feel really good. Linger in that feel-good state as you think about that one best thing that happened today. Tell yourself you did a great job today.

Say a thank you for the quality sleep you will have, and recite an affirmation, such as "All is well in my life."

Aim to live in a healthier state of being, one that is helpful, nourishing, and uplifting for all aspects of our life. Learn to choose love and all its related feelings over fear and all of its related feelings. Learn to take responsibility for the energy and attitude you choose to give in each and every moment. This is a huge part of keeping your body and mind fit, healthy, and strong.

Blessings-consciousness keeps us in a state of appreciation.

Appreciation is a powerful, life-changing energy when practiced all day every day. It is a form of love and peace, and it moves from your spirit self instead of your ego self. It is available to you every moment of your life, regardless of the circumstances and situations you find yourself in. **You can always find something to appreciate right now, no matter what.** It is just a matter of where you decide to put your focus and attention.

Right now, find something you can say "thank you" for. Look at everything going on in your life through the eyes of appreciation. Focus on everything and everyone in your life you are grateful for. Don't stop this focus until you start feeling better. Every person, every moment, everything is a gift, even the challenging people and moments. They are in your life for the experience, so that you can learn and grow as a person. List your appreciations mentally or write them down. Feel the feeling of thankfulness. Say, "Thank you." I usually feel a warm, tingly sensation when I mentally focus on all that I appreciate. It's like God is hugging me and saying, "You are welcome." Again, this one practice shifted my life. It wasn't forced, and it wasn't work; it was a sincere practice, a committed choice to go through my day appreciating everything and everyone. This attitude brings an immediate calm, lightness, and ease to your being, which then gets radiated outward into your world.

Why practice blessings-consciousness and appreciation?

Appreciation is an expression of love. Appreciation helps you focus on what's going well, what's good and right in your life instead of dwelling on what's wrong, what's not happening fast enough, and what you want to be different.

Appreciation helps you be abundance-minded, instead of lack-minded. Our blessings are multiplied because what we focus on expands, and our loving universe gives us more of what we focus on.

Appreciation creates a feeling of joy and happiness within us, which is then felt by everyone and everything around us. The energy of appreciation is the energy of love, and it draws more and more things we love into our lives. Appreciation puts us in a state of calmness and contentment right here and right now. These are healthy states for your body to be in.

Appreciation **instantly** shifts our energy from negative to positive when practiced in the moment. When we live with appreciation, fear cannot enter. You cannot feel appreciation and any negative emotion at the same time.

When appreciating through challenges and problems, you are able to remain calm, clear-minded, and focused, so solutions can come to you more readily than in a state of worry or fear. **You cannot be in a state of appreciation and worry or fear at the same time.**

Acknowledging the good that you already have in your life is the foundation for all abundance.
—Eckhart Tolle

Are you struggling with something or someone in your life? **Do not allow yourself to linger in negativity. Do not allow yourself to linger in a victim mentality.** Work through your situations putting your best self forward. I know we all go through times when we feel overwhelmed by so much happening at once, and so many things need our attention. It's important to keep in mind that we are never given more than we can handle. There's an ebb and flow to life. Do your best to ride it out and work it out by always keeping in mind the things you can control and change, and allowing everything and everyone else to be.

We each have our own journey to walk. You can't walk another person's journey for them. You can encourage and inspire, but ultimately you need to allow others to experience their own choices, just as you experience yours. Someone hurt you so much that sending them good thoughts is a stretch for you right now? Then, at the very least, choose not to send them negative thoughts or talk about them negatively by criticizing, condemning, judging, or complaining. Let them be. Let God and the universe handle the situation. You just control *you*.

Do your best not to take other people's actions personally. We create so much stress and drama within ourselves when we imagine the worst, take on other people's problems, or take bad treatment personally. The other person is feeling pain, hurt, and unhappiness, and they don't know what to do with that pain, so they dish it out. Just bless them with healing love and prayers. This is sometimes the best way to resolve an issue with someone who's challenging and you don't seem to get anywhere with verbal communication. Take the optimistic approach and send them good thoughts. Sending love and goodness is nourishing and helpful. Sending negative thoughts and energy to someone or a situation only hurts you. Keep yourself in check and practice optimism. Don't engage in negativity. If someone is deliberately pushing your buttons, walk away. Keep calm and walk away. It is never about you. Sometimes the only thing you can do is disengage from them entirely and send good thoughts and prayers, at least for now.

Make a commitment to approach every situation and circumstance as a blessing for you, even those things that seem to be tough and hard to face, and those events that don't turn out the way you had planned. Hold some space for trust in life and the universe. Keeping your attention and focus on blessings-consciousness allows you to stay connected to your spirit, which is a healthy and happy place to be and live.

> *For God did not give us a spirit of timidity, but*
> *a spirit of power, love and self-discipline.*
> **—2 Timothy 1:7**

Two: Practice Optimism

Now that you are developing a habit of focusing on your blessings, bring a state of optimism to each and every situation and circumstance you're experiencing. Optimism is an attitude.

The dictionary describes optimism as a commitment to look on the more favorable side of events, situations, and conditions. **To expect a favorable outcome**. What you expect, you get. So, what are you expecting? Be hopeful that everything will always turn out for your benefit. Sometimes when we're going through a hard time, it's tough to stay positive. But you can choose to stay optimistic. You can choose to discipline your mind to see the good in all situations. When we discipline our minds to view everything in an optimistic way, our thoughts will remain optimistic. Our conversations will remain optimistic. Our actions will be optimistic. We will be in a state of calmness, lightness, and ease, which keeps our body healthy, fit, and strong. You can't be negative and optimistic at the same time. You get to choose. One choice is toxic to the body, and the other is healthy. Optimism keeps you in a state of hope. Never give up hope!

Practicing optimism is choosing to refuse to allow outside circumstances and situations to affect you negatively. Developing optimism requires disciplining your mind to expect a good outcome. Everything starts in your mind; whatever you expect, you will experience. By consciously choosing to keep an optimistic attitude no matter what's going on around us, we gain greater strength and control over our emotional state of mind. **We don't have to allow outer circumstances to affect us negatively.** We **always** have a choice as to how we will respond and perceive a situation. The health of our physical body will be affected by what we choose. Be diligent in disciplining yourself to speak only words that are uplifting, nourishing, and helpful to yourself and all aspects of your life. This is the simplest way to stay optimistic. **Watch what you say and how you say it.** If you have nothing good to say about someone or something, be silent.

An optimistic attitude keeps you motivated to move forward in a helpful way. Staying in a state of optimism keeps you calm and focused. When you are calm and focused, new ideas and plans come to you more easily than if you are in a state of worry and anxiety. New opportunities and people will come into your life that are helpful and encouraging for you. You may think it's luck or a coincidence, but it's really your optimistic state of mind and energy attracting positive circumstances. Choose to focus on a positive outcome. Instead of worry and fear, which is toxic to the body when lingered over a period of time, visualize and expect a good outcome. If you find yourself nervous or stressed, take a timeout, breathe, and recite a positive affirmation. When you linger in optimism, no matter what, you will end up attracting opportunities, people, events, and circumstances that are helpful for your growth and success. Deliberately choose to project this energy out in the world, and experience your goodness!

The simplest way I have found to practice optimism is to set your intention each morning that no matter what you are doing, or where you need to be, you will choose to see the positive, you will choose to expect a good outcome, and you will choose to see the good in everyone and everything. That's it—simple, but not always easy.

So what are you expecting? Are you expecting things to work out for your benefit? As you expect, so it will be for you.

Three: Practice Meditation

Be still, and know that I am God.
—Psalm 46:10

Our breath is a blessing. Don't underestimate the power of your breath to immediately bring your body and mind calmness and peace. Mediation is a practice aimed to calm the ongoing chatter of the mind, which is usually negative and generates all sorts of stressful feelings and pain in our body.

As explained by Sri Ramana Maharshi, "Meditation is sticking to one thought. That thought keeps away other thoughts; distraction of the mind is a sign of its weakness; by constant meditation it gains strength."

Benefits of Meditation

- Calms the body and mind
- Reduces stress and anxiety
- Has healing benefits for the body by normalizing blood pressure
- Brings calmness to others around a person who meditates

- Improves your ability to focus and concentrate
- Improves the ability to stay present in your life
- Brings about happiness, contentment, and a state of ease
- Brings about a spiritual awakening
- Decreases victim mentality
- Reduces inflammation in the body

Now, don't you want to reap the results of meditation? Start now, and don't complicate this!

Taking a 5–10 minute timeout to deliberately breathe deeply and consciously is one the most calming things you can do. Five minutes to pull yourself together when you feel a bit unraveled. Don't underestimate the power of your breath. It's your key to calmness, wellness, and good health—instantly. Negative feelings dissipate quickly when you deliberately take a timeout for conscious breathing. **Using your breath immediately brings you back to your present moment.**

Tips for Practicing Meditation

- Meditate every day.
- Stay in an optimistic attitude. Refuse to entertain any thoughts that you can't do it, or it's a waste of time, or you don't have time for it, or you can't stop your thoughts. You're not trying to stop your thoughts; you're just calming your thoughts down a bit and training your mind to focus.
- Meditate in a quiet place and where you can be alone.
- Sit straight up on your "sit bones," back straight, shoulders relaxed and down.
- Start breathing slowly.
- Set a timer for five or ten minutes

My personal practice is as follows: I inhale deeply and say, "Thank you, God." I hold my breath for a moment. I exhale completely and repeat, "All is well in my life, and everything is unfolding as it should."

You can use whatever positive affirmation works for you during your breathing. The possibilities are endless. Use what feels right to you. Just make sure it's positive, calming, and present tense.

When breathing, use what is called "ocean breath." When breathing this way, it sounds like the ocean. This instantly energizes you, rejuvenates you, and brings clarity and focus back to the present moment. Go ahead and make an ocean sound with your breath as you breathe in and out. You will hear the ocean in your breath. Try breathing in and out with your mouth closed. If you can't get the ocean sound, then breath with your mouth open and then try to close it.

Besides focusing your mind on an affirmation, you can choose to focus your mind on an object, such as a candle or a mental image, such as the ocean. You can focus your mind on music or just focus on your breathing.

This personal practice brings me a state of peace, calmness, and serenity. Try mine or develop your own.

There are many guided meditations available to you, and even meditation classes. Whatever you choose, just start and do it. It will change your life. There is no wrong way to meditate. Just start. Stay with it and enjoy the results of your efforts!

Meditation is a spiritual practice. I consider prayer a type of meditation. Praying daily keeps me connected to God. Ballroom dancing is also a practice that connects me to my spirit that I love to do. Doing things I love to do keeps me connected to God. What do you love to do? When you are happy, when you give love and do the things you love to do in life, that's your greatest gift to God, who has blessed you with this beautiful journey called life. Stay connected. Meditate, pray, love, and do the things you love to do in life.

There are many ways to connect to your spirit and be with God.

I have a brother who loves to hunt. I am convinced that the only reason he does it is to sit in silence in the dark and just be. He loves to sit in a tree, in the woods, at 3:00 in the morning. That is his type of spiritual connection. He is silent. He is in nature.

I have a sister who prays the rosary every morning. That is her chosen spiritual daily practice that keeps her connected with God and starts her day from her spirit.

My mom goes to church every Sunday and has done so each and every Sunday ever since I can remember.

Meditate, pray, and do the things you love to do. Develop a spiritual practice—whatever that means to you, and doing whatever nourishes you. It's different for everyone and evolves and grows. Maybe you had a foundation of Catholicism or Buddhism, and your spiritual journey led you elsewhere. Go with it. It is **your** spiritual journey, and if it is nourishing, helpful, loving, and uplifting, it is from God, and it is good.

Get into the habit of giving yourself a mental and emotional **timeout** when you start feeling any negative emotion. When you start to feel anger, frustration, impatience, anxiety, whatever, **stop**. Take a minute or two and just start breathing deeply and intentionally, and repeat an "I am calm" or "I am at peace" or "Let it go." Disciplining yourself this way creates calm and centeredness. This timeout gives us greater control of our feelings and emotions, restores our peace and serenity, and keeps our stress level under control. If starting a meditation just seems too much for you, at the very least, practice taking peaceful timeouts when you need to. After two minutes, ask yourself, "What is the most helpful, nourishing, and uplifting thing I can do, say, or think right now?"

Four: Do Something Nourishing, Helpful, and Uplifting

Hit your happy list and engage fully in an activity that nourishes and uplifts you. This is an action step. Move toward your goals. Engage fully in an activity that will help you feel better. This will shift your energy to a better place. Doing something physical gets the tension and stress out of your body and calms your mind.

- Take a walk outside.
- Go for a run.
- Hike in the woods.
- Sit by the lake or beach.
- Take an exercise class.
- Put some music on and dance.
- Watch a comedy.
- Meditate.
- Pet your dog/cat.
- Listen to soothing music.
- Pray.
- Write in a journal. Write a letter.
- Write out positive affirmations.
- Call someone who is supportive, positive, encouraging, and helpful.
- Donate time to a charity.
- Do a puzzle or play a board game, ping pong, chess, paint, etc.
- Step away from the computer, phone, news, etc. and give yourself a disconnect.
- Spend time with uplifting and nourishing people you enjoy.
- Explore and experience wellness therapies. Massage therapy, acupuncture, Reiki, Rolfing, tai chi, qigong, homeopathic medicine, and reflexology are just a few wellness therapies that have been shown to improve health and well-being.

Take action. Do something that puts your mind in a healthy place. That shifts your emotions to a calmer place.

This action step needs to be a nourishing, helpful, and uplifting choice. Using food, alcohol, drugs, or any other addictive substance is not nourishing, helpful, or uplifting. These are numbing choices, and it leads to experiencing a consequence you probably don't want to experience.

Set time aside for doing something you enjoy. Do you know what you enjoy doing? Are you making time for these activities that feed your spirit?

> *All effort must be made by you.*
> **—Buddha**

Five: Practice Allowance and Acceptance

Say "yes" to life, and say "yes" to your present moment. Trust that all is always well and that life is unfolding as it should. There are no accidents. There are no coincidences.

When we have done our best in thoughts, words, actions, and attitudes, we can await the results in peace. We all want things the way we want them, and we want people to be and act the way we want them to, and we want our bodies to change yesterday from the healthy effort we have made, and we want results *right now*. Well, we have to grow up and be patient and allow life to unfold. God's timing may not be the same as our timing. Do and be your best, and allow the results to be. What will be, will be; we can only control what we can.

Affirm daily: "I will do and be my best today, and allow everything and everyone else to be." "All is well in my life. I will allow this day, this moment, to be." "My life is unfolding as it should."

Always keep in mind that you can only change and be in control of you. Acceptance is allowing life to unfold and trusting that all is well—always. It is about choosing faith and trust. Choose to trust the process of life, and refuse to allow any doubt to enter into your energy. Sometimes it's easier to feel what "not allowing" is in order to know "allowing."

Not Allowing = Resistance

Resisting the moment is the cause of **all** fear, worry, stress, anger, etc. It is the cause of **all** pain. It's a state of wanting things to be different and trying to control things and people that you have no control over. What you resist will persist in your life. You need to just make the commitment to do and be the best you can with what you know right now, with where you are and what you have, and *allow life to unfold*. I can guarantee if you're feeling stressed, worried, afraid, or any other negative emotion, it is because you're resisting something going on. When you release resistance, you allow wellness.

Remember, you cannot have a negative emotion and be in a state of allowing at the same time. You cannot radiate an uplifting, nourishing energy and a negative energy at the same time. You get to choose, and it's always your choice no matter what's going on.

*If you knew **who** walks beside you … fear would be impossible.*
—A Course in Miracles

Allow other people, including your loved ones, to experience the choices they make. Refrain from complaining about others and let go of the need to change people and situations that bug you. This is so important in order to keep a state of peace within yourself. This is also very hard to do sometimes. You can reach out with good intentions, in love, kindness, and compassion, and be the healthiest and happiest example you can be, but **you cannot change anyone. You can only change yourself**. This is such an important part of allowing, and one that I work on daily. I want to help *everyone* be healthy and happy, but you can't force it. People have to live their own lives and experience their own choices, including those you love. If you assume responsibility for other people, no matter who it is, you will be overwhelmed, resentful, and angry, feel drained and tired, and experience all kinds of physical problems from headaches to digestive issues to pain in your muscles. Understand that focusing on changing and controlling *you* is not selfish. It's actually the opposite. **When you get healthier, happier, and content, the world enjoys you more.** The best gift you can give your loved ones is to **be as happy and healthy as you can** and hold them up in the most uplifted, optimistic, and helpful way in your prayers and thoughts. Let them work through their "stuff," and you tend to your own. **Trust the process of life to take care of you and your loved ones.**

Give your attention and focus to what is important to you. It is impossible to change another person. The sooner you accept that, the more you free up your energy and time to do the things that are important to you. You can only change and control *your* thoughts and actions, how *you* speak, and the attitude *you* bring to each moment of the day. These choices create your life, no matter what anyone else is thinking or doing. Mind your own life.

Always remember that we are all spiritual beings having a very *human* experience. We have all made mistakes, mistreated loved ones, and acted in ways that aren't uplifting, helpful, and nourishing. If you have a person in your life that is a challenge for you, **thank them** for teaching you how to love them anyway. Allow them to be who and what they want to be, and hold them up in your thoughts and prayers. Remember, **what you give, is what you get**. So, give uplifting, nourishing thoughts and words about all others, including those that challenge you—even if you feel justified in your anger and resentment. That justification will hold you in a victim mode, and you will experience more circumstances to justify your anger and resentment. **Break out of it** by thinking differently. If someone isn't loving and caring to themselves or the person closest to them, how can you expect them to be loving and caring to you? If they are mistreating and disrespecting their body with alcohol, drugs, excess food, or not enough food, how can you expect them to be treating you with respect? People can only give what they can. If they're not feeling good about themselves, they won't be treating themselves well. If they're not treating themselves well, they're not going to treat others well. Control and change what you can.

Allowance requires patience. Allowance requires letting go. Letting go means just stopping. Just stop. Detach. Go with the flow and allow life to unfold. Be in a state of calmness. Keep your mind and body in a state of ease. It is not giving up. It is choosing to move into your world from a place of ease, trust, and love instead of anxiety, fear, and anger. Breathe and let it be. Let life be. We want our way right now. We want our results right now. We want, we want, we want, and we want it right now. Just stop. Breathe and let it be. Stop blaming, stop condemning, stop criticizing, stop arguing, stop wishing things were different, stop being a victim, and stop trying to control and manipulate other people in order to change them. **Just stop—breathe—and let it be.** When we finally do stop, we experience peace and calmness, we are less tense, and we are clear-minded enough to change something that we can control.

Learning to practice acceptance in our relationships helps us maintain a peaceful state of mind. If we are in disagreement with someone, it is usually because we feel frustrated with our inability to change the circumstance or change the person. Understanding we can only change and control ourselves in the way we think, talk, behave, and the attitude we give, we let go of our expectations of others and focus on ourselves. This empowers you because you start to realize that your own inner peace does not depend upon anyone or anything but your own state of mind.

Practicing acceptance and the other choose-well steps releases negative, toxic thoughts and feelings from the body. Working out and sweating releases toxins and stress. Drinking enough water releases toxins. All these forms of release and letting go are so helpful for keeping your body and mind fit, healthy and strong.

Trust in the Lord with all your heart; lean not on your own understanding. In all your ways acknowledge him and he shall direct thy path.
—Proverbs 3:5-6

Wrap-Up

Choosing nourishing, uplifting, and helpful thoughts, attitudes, words, and actions is extremely important for living a healthy and happy life. Having a victim mentality is the number-one reason you get in your own way of reaching your goals and dreams, and it's toxic to the physical body. Research has shown that lingering in negative thoughts and feelings has a toxic effect on the body, and stress is the cause of 99 percent of all diseases known to man.

Stop criticizing, complaining, condemning, blaming, gossiping, judging, and being angry, resentful, and guilty. Stop the victim mentality and own your power to choose.

Use the five choose-well lifestyle practices to manage your state of mind and emotions. Count your blessings and live in a state of appreciation, practice optimism, practice meditation, take action to shift into a better-feeling state, and practice allowing and accepting the moment.

Pay attention to your attitude, your behavior, and your conversations. Keep in mind the two choose-well questions: "What am I choosing to give?" And "Is this choice nourishing, uplifting, and helpful?" Asking yourself questions and listening for the answer keeps you **aware** and **living in the present moment**. It also gives you the opportunity to decide if you want to experience the result of the choice you are making.

Make a commitment to practice the next four fundamentals to create a fit, healthy, strong body and state of mind!

Suggested Reading :
Any book from Louise Hay, Wayne Dwyer, Alan
Cohen, Eckhart Tolle, or Guy Finley
Happy Pocket Full of Money by David Cameron Gikandi
The Law of Attraction by Esther and Jerry Hicks
Integrative Nutrition by Joshua Rosenthal
The Dynamic Laws of Prosperity by Catherine Ponder

FUNDAMENTAL TWO: KEEP IT CLEAN

WHATEVER YOU PUT in your mouth, keep it clean. Whether it is food or liquids, make healthy, clean choices to create a fit, healthy, strong body and state of mind. You have probably heard this a million times, but I'm going to mention it here anyway. You are what you eat. And you can also say, you are what you think and do. Every cell in our body is breaking down and rebuilding, and the state of health your cells rebuild themselves with is directly determined by what you choose to eat, drink, do, and think. Take a look at someone who eats plenty of lean protein, whole grains, fruits, vegetables, nuts, and seeds, and you will most likely observe someone with a positive, radiant glow of good health and well-being. Observe a fast-food, junk-food junkie, and you will most likely see someone who is moody, tired, overweight, cranky, and puffy looking.

No single food will make or break good health. But the kinds of food you choose day in and day out have a major impact.
—Walter Willet, MD

Eating clean, whole foods is a simple practice. It may not always be easy or convenient, but it is simple. Does it take a commitment? Yes. Does it take planning? Yes. Does it take mindfulness? Yes. But making the choice to commit, plan, and be mindful is worth the results you will experience.

Why do we eat foods we know we should avoid? Why do we eat portions that we know are too large? Why are the fast-food restaurants always full of people? Why do we eat junk food, fast food, processed food, high-fat and high-calorie food and think it's weird to drink wheat grass? So many factors influence our eating habits, from social pressure, to heredity, to economics, to convenience. **The bottom line is that no matter what, it's your choices that are creating the health of your physical body, and it's going to mean cleaning up those choices to reap a healthier result.** So, start where you are and clean up what needs to be cleaned up. It's up to you to choose nourishing foods. Start right now, where you are. It's never too late to clean up your eating habits. All you have to do is choose to start. **Right now.**

There are many diet plans that help you lose weight with prepackaged foods. Again, even though these plans "work" and help you lose weight, they're not the healthiest because all prepackaged foods are processed with preservatives. **I am promoting and encouraging clean-food eating. Nature's goodness. One-ingredient foods.**

Food-related disease combined with a sedentary lifestyle is the number-one cause of preventable death. The obesity rate is staggering in this country, and our health care system is overloaded. We spend two trillion dollars per year on health care, and we are becoming more and more unhealthy. Our kids are now becoming pre-diabetic. The only way to help this situation is **on an individual basis; we need to decide to take responsibility for our lifestyle and eating habits.** We need to pull ourselves together and make more choices that are nourishing for our bodies. Our society may be overweight, but we are nutritionally starving. Our society eats too much refined carbohydrates, too much fast food, too much sugar, and too much processed and packaged foods. And to top that off, we tend to go for the latest and greatest fad and craze to lose weight quickly. It is insane. It is unhealthy, and it does more harm than good in the long run for your body. You have to decide whether you want wellness or sickness. Your choice.

THE CHOOSE-WELL EATING PLAN

Suggested attitude focus: Shift your attitude and focus from "weight loss" to "being healthy." Stop dieting and start eating for a fit, healthy, strong body and state of mind.

Why? You will **allow** your body to change to a healthier state without getting in your own way with your negative thinking and attitude. If you have some weight to lose, no matter how much it is, you didn't put the weight on overnight, and you won't lose it overnight. Allow yourself to succeed. Shifting your attitude from weight loss to being healthy will also allow you to practice patience with your body, and it gives you the opportunity to focus on all the other amazing health benefits that eating well and exercising have on your life. **Fad diets do not work.** Get back to nature's goodness. Good health and well-being are about more than a number on a scale and more than getting skinny. A healthy, strong, and nourished body is rarely bloated, fatigued, and feeling heavy. When your physical body is fit and strong, you *feel* fit and strong. You feel agile, energized, and happy. Understand some of us are naturally thin, and some of us are naturally curvy. Embrace the genetics given to you, and be as healthy and happy as you can be. No matter what our genetic state may be, we can all make a commitment to being healthy in mind, attitude, and body, and release the "skinny" wish that causes all sorts of stress, anxiety, self-loathing, and a give-up attitude. When your body is physically healthy and strong, your mind will be clear and focused.

Suggested food focus: keep it clean with high fiber and healthy fat nourishment.

The choose-well plan is about crowding out the junk with good, clean, natural fibrous foods. Along with a fiber focus is a healthy fat focus, specifically foods rich in super-healthy omega-3 fatty acids. **Fiber, healthy fats, and water make a perfect combination!**

Let's chat about carbs. **Carbohydrates are not your enemy.** Fast food, processed food, junk food, and packaged food are your body's enemy. Carbohydrates are necessary for the body to function efficiently. Fibrous carbohydrates found in fruits, vegetables, legumes, and whole grains are you body's powerhouse. They provide fuel for the body, giving you abundant energy, and they provide fiber. You need carbs not only for energy, but to ensure your brain and nervous system function well, and to help the body use fat efficiently. Think of carbs as your energy nutrient.

A case for fiber: I don't think it's a coincidence that we eat on average ten grams of fiber per day, and this country is getting fatter and fatter and sicker and sicker. Then we turn to pharmaceuticals with all the awful side effects, without taking a look at our eating habits, lack of exercise, or emotional state. I also don't think there is a soul out there that will dispute the fact that if we increase our intake of fruits, vegetables, legumes, beans, nuts, and whole grains, and decrease out intake of processed packaged foods and fast foods, we will create a much healthier country, and our health care system may start to get out of the crisis it is in.

No matter what controversy surrounds food and nutrition, one fact remains consistent. **A high-fiber, clean diet leads to brilliant health and well-being.** We need to get back to basics, and the simplest way to do that is to make sure you get a minimum of twenty-five grams of fiber per day. Why? What are the positive consequences of a diet rich in fiber? They are: healthy digestive system; healthy immune system; prevents obesity and weight gain; fills you up and stabilizes blood-sugar levels for hours; tames your appetite; fiber-rich foods aren't as calorie dense, so you can fill up on high-fiber foods but take in fewer calories; increases your energy, gives you better sleep, and increases your mental well-being and focus. Who doesn't want to reap those results!

3 Steps to a Healthy Meal

1. Choose your fiber and aim for 8 grams (fruits, veggies, whole grains, nuts, legumes)
2. Choose your healthy anti-inflammatory fat in at least two of the meals (nuts, olive oil, avocado, chia   seeds, flax seed, wild-caught salmon, etc.).
3. Choose your lean protein.

*Aim for 25–35 grams of fiber per day—8 grams per meal, 4 grams per snack. Have three meals per day, and one or two snacks per day.

Breakfast/Lunch/Dinner

Divide your plate into three portions. Half your plate is your veggie/fruit portion, a quarter of your plate is your high-fiber, complex whole grain carb portion, and a quarter of your plate is your lean protein portion.

Eyeball your portions. The palm of your hand is your protein portion. Have a big (two open palms, cupped hand) green-veggie portion and other colorful veggies. One open palm (cupped hand) is your whole-grain portion (between a half and one cup, or two slices of high-fiber bread). Have one piece of fruit.

For snacks, have one piece of fruit and one serving of nuts.

So, choose your lean protein. Be mindful of your portion. Choose your high-fiber carb. Be mindful of your portion. Choose your fruit and/or vegetable/leafy green. Choose your omega-3 healthy fat. Be mindful of your portion. **Eat slowly.** Repeat for each meal.

Sample Breakfast Choices

1 cup Greek plain yogurt, 1 tablespoon chia seeds, 1 serving of whole grain granola/cereal, 1 cup berries
1 cup steel cut oats, 1 tablespoon chia seeds, 1 apple
Smoothie (1 cup coconut water, 1 cup of water, 1 banana, 1 scoop protein powder, 2 tablespoons ground flaxseed, 1 tablespoon of wheat grass)

Sample Lunch Choices

Leafy greens, sliced carrots, cucumbers, ½ cup chick peas, 1 serving grilled chicken. Olive oil/vinegar dressing.
2 slices of whole grain bread, 2 tablespoons nut butter, 1 tablespoon chia seeds, 1 pear
1 whole grain wrap, sliced fresh turkey, ¼ of avocado, sliced tomatoes, and lettuce. 1 cup cherries

Sample Dinner Choices

Grilled shrimp, sautéed kale (cooked in a
little olive oil), ½ cup quinoa
Roasted salmon, ½ cup brown rice, sautéed broccoli rabe
Baked chicken, steamed broccoli, ½ cup quinoa
1 cup lentils, ½ cup whole grain pasta, 2 tablespoons
grated cheese. Green salad with olive oil dressing.

Each meal has a lean protein choice, high-fiber whole grain choice, fruit/vegetable choice, and a healthy fat omega-3 choice. Each meal has at least eight grams of fiber.

Do your best to make your fiber choice whole, clean foods made from nature and not man. If you choose breads, cereals, bars, and pastas or anything else packaged, make sure it has a good amount of fiber, has a minimum number of ingredients, and is made of ingredients that you can understand when you read the label.

Counting Your Fiber Grams (roughly, on average)

Beans, ½ cup = 8 grams of fiber
Veggies, 1 cup = 4 grams of fiber
Leafy greens, one cup = 2 grams of fiber
Fruit, one piece = 3 grams of fiber
Whole grains (brown rice, whole grain pasta,
oatmeal, quinoa, etc.) = 4 grams per serving
Nuts, one serving, ¼ cup = 3 grams of fiber
Flaxseed, 2 tablespoons = 4 grams of fiber
Chia seeds, 2 tablespoons = 8 grams of fiber
Meat, dairy, seafood, fish, poultry = 0 grams of fiber

Suggested Practice: For one month, actively and intentionally count your fiber grams using whole, clean food choices, and I can guarantee you will feel healthy, energized, and even lose a few pounds. After one month of counting, you will have developed a habit of eating clean and healthy foods and won't have to count anymore. It's just a part of your healthy lifestyle now.

How much fiber are you getting a day? Keep a food journal and actively count your fiber grams. Starting with breakfast, increase your intake and work from them. Aim to have a high-fiber breakfast each morning for a week, and then start focusing on lunch for a week. And then move to dinner for a week. After three weeks, you will be amazed how your body and mind feel!

Surround your meals and snacks with plenty of green, colorful vegetables, fruits, nuts, legumes, and whole grains. Filling up on fibrous foods will keep you feeling satisfied, curb cravings, and you will not have room in your belly for junk. It is that simple.

Top Fiber Foods—Nature's Goodness

Wholesome Grains: One of the easiest ways to increase your fiber intake is to focus on whole grains. A whole grain is a grain in its natural state—nothing processed, nothing left out. When a grain is refined (as in lots of packaged foods), the germ and the bran are removed. In other words, all the "goodness" of the grain is removed, resulting in fiber, protein and other nutrients lost. Some excellent examples of whole grains are: Oats, barley, air popped popcorn, quinoa, brown rice, oat bran, wheat bran, millet, barely, wild rice, whole wheat pasta.

Beans and Legumes: From frozen to fresh, canned to dried, peas and beans are one of the most natural, rich sources of fiber, protein, vitamins, and minerals. A true super-food. Whether enjoying a nourishing bowl of lentils or tossing them in a salad, a serving of beans per day is a must, in my opinion. Loaded with nourishment, some great examples are black beans, green peas, spilt peas, lentils, garbanzo beans, white/navy/kidney beans, and lima beans.

Berries: Although berries are a fruit, I am listing them separately because of the high fiber content of certain berries. Blackberries and raspberries have eight grams of fiber per one cup serving! Strawberries and blueberries have four grams per one cup.

Nuts and Seeds: One ounce of nuts, about a handful or a quarter cup, provides a hearty contribution to the day's fiber count. It's a great afternoon snack with a piece of fruit! Another bonus of nuts is that they provide healthy fats and a good dose of protein. Examples include almonds, pistachio nuts, peanuts/cashews/walnuts, sunflower seeds, ground flaxseed, and sesame seed.

Dark, Leafy Greens: Oh what a super, super food leafy greens are! Enjoy two large servings of greens per day for super-duper nourishment. Rich in beta carotene, vitamins, and minerals, they supply a good dose of fiber. Enjoy a big green salad and a generous serving of sautéed greens in a little olive oil, lemon, and garlic. Turnip/mustard/collard greens, spinach, Swiss chard, salad greens, kale, broccoli, Brussels sprouts, and cabbage are all excellent choices.

Potatoes: Although they sometimes get a bad rap, the potato itself is a healthy food. It's what you put on top of it that gets you in trouble. And although it's a "white" food, it's a whole food with fiber and nutrients. A russet potato (with skin) has four grams of fiber, a red potato (with skin) has three grams, and a nourishing sweet potato (with skin) has four grams.

Fruit Basket: What a healthy habit to get into to reach for an apple, a pear, or an orange as a snack. Keep fresh fruit readily available. Fruit is naturally packed with fiber, vitamins, and minerals. Most pieces of fruit have about three grams of fiber, although a pear packs about six grams!

Again, although fiber is added to almost anything, I highly encourage nature-made food instead of man-made food!

It takes an intention to want to eat well. It takes planning, planning, and planning to support this intention. Just stay in the moment and choose the best you can. Have fun with this. Choose to nourish yourself with clean, whole foods out of love and respect for yourself.

A Brief Chat about Protein

Think of protein as your building and repairing nutrient. Protein is a nutrient found in food that builds and repairs body tissue. It is the major component of enzymes, hormones, and antibodies. Protein is not a major source of energy; it is simply used by the body to build and repair muscles, ligaments, and tendons. The simplest way to make sure you are getting enough protein in your daily intake is to have a portioned serving of a lean, clean protein at each meal. **Lean and clean** is the emphasis. Combining a lean protein and a high-fiber carb makes for a satisfying, nourishing, and energy-producing combination.

Any animal protein should be no bigger than the size of the palm of your hand. This choice makes up a quarter of your plate at breakfast, lunch, and dinner. If chicken is your choice, organic would be the cleanest, healthiest choice. If beef is your choice, grass fed would be the cleanest choice. Eat a variety of lean meats, fish, and seafood to keep your body healthy. Baked, broiled, poached, grilled, and roasted are the leanest ways of preparing.

Eating too much animal protein has been shown to cause lots of health problem, especially in those overweight and sedentary. Cutting back may be the choice for you. Try to go a few days without meat. Choose fish and seafood or beans and tofu, along with your veggies and whole grains, and then journal how you feel. I personally need animal protein in my nutritional plan to keep me grounded and feeling my best.

Healthy animal proteins include organic poultry, lean cuts of pork loin, grass-fed range beef, eggs, fish, seafood, and shellfish. Have a variety of fish and seafood choices to reduce the mercury levels taken in.

Low-fat dairy choices include low-fat milk, skim milk, plain yogurt, cottage cheese, plain Greek yogurt, and non-processed real cheese.

Vegetarian protein choices include all kinds of beans and legumes, tofu and edamame. Read labels carefully when purchasing processed tofu products. These are still processed foods and not the cleanest or the healthiest.

Experiment with protein. Try to go meat-free for a week. Pay attention to how you feel and journal it. Do you feel more energized, clear-minded, and focused? Does your body feel cleaner and less bloated and tired? Or do you feel a little scattered and hungry?

Healthy Fats

Let's talk healthy fats. Fat provides the chief storage of energy in the body, provides insulation and protection of vital organs, and provides fat-soluble vitamins. Omega-3s are the healthy fats and vital to good health for your mind and body. These fatty acids help your skin and hair look and feel healthy, keep your cells working properly, and decrease inflammation in the body. Think of healthy fats as an anti-inflammatory for your body, which is why I suggest making sure you eat enough omega-3 rich foods in your daily meal plan. Just a little goes a long way.

Healthy fats include almonds, walnuts, sunflower seeds, olives, olive oil, avocados, avocado oil, flaxseed, and cashews.

Omega-3 rich foods include flaxseeds, chia seeds, walnuts, wild-caught salmon, sardines, soybeans, halibut, scallops, shrimp, tofu, tuna, spinach, collard greens, kale, squash, cod, green beans, miso, strawberries, Brussels sprouts, raspberries, eggs, and grass-fed meat.

When you combine the anti-inflammatory benefits of omega-3 rich foods with the health benefits of fiber-rich food, you have a super-healthy combination to help you create a fit, strong, and healthy body and mind!

This is a very brief overview of healthy and nourishing eating. We can go on and on about food, what to eat, what not to eat, and quite honestly, I think it makes for more and more confusion. **Keep it simple. Focus on nature's goodness.** Have fun being in the driver's seat of your eating plan and figuring out what works well for your body and what doesn't.

Some Additional Suggestions

Cook your own food instead of going out to eat. Why? You know what's in your food, how it's cooked, and you put your love and energy into cooking it. Have you ever gone into a restaurant, and the energy of the people working there, or even the people dining there was not positive, calm, and nurturing? Did you feel sick after eating, or the day after? You are taking in the energy of the people around your food and preparing your food.

Say thank you before eating. Take a breath, sit down, plate your food, engage in no other activity, and say, "Thank you for nourishing my body."

Eat slowly. I can't stress this enough. Chew your food well. Digestion starts in the mouth. All sorts of digestive problems can be solved by just chewing your food slowly. Slowing your eating down helps your digestive system stay healthy, your body absorbs nutrients better, and you enjoy your meal so much more. Try chewing twenty times before swallowing. You will even find yourself eating less if you just slow down!

Stop eating before you feel full. I know some of us are used to cleaning our plates. Get out of that habit. Practice listening to your body and recognize the feeling of being almost full and just stop. Eat when you are hungry, not starving, and stop when your stomach feels *almost* full.

Drink less alcohol. Even though studies have suggested that moderate alcohol (one drink per day for women, two for men) has some healthy benefits like raising good HDL cholesterol, there are also reasons to keep alcohol consumption to moderation. It takes a toll on the liver, which is the body's major organ to detox your system, it acts as a diuretic so it's harder to stay hydrated, and it adds liquid calories to your daily calorie intake. My clients dropped significant weight when they made the choice to drink less alcohol.

Cut back on salt. Americans eat an average of 3,400 milligrams of sodium in a day. That is 1,000 mg more than we should be taking in. Making a choice to cut back 1,000 mg per day would lower the risk of heart disease by 9 percent. Restaurant foods, fast food, and processed foods tend to be very high in sodium. Choose to eat out less, cook at home, and eat less processed/packaged foods.

Eat less sugar. On average, Americans consume 475 calories of added sugar per day—that's thirty teaspoons. Go ahead and spoon out thirty teaspoons of sugar to get a visual of that. Yikes. High intake of sugar is linked to all sorts of disease in the body, from cancer to heart disease to high triglyceride levels in the blood. Reach for your fruit bowl when wanting something sweet and skip the processed/packaged foods.

Eat less refined grains and processed foods. Processed and packaged foods with lots of ingredients listed are loaded with added sugar, added salt, and saturated fats. Skip the chips and crackers and go for the fresh veggies and popcorn.

GETTING STARTED

Keep a food journal. Write everything down—how much you eat, why you are eating, how you feel as you are eating, how you feel when you are done eating. Write down everything you are drinking, including water intake. Writing down your food and beverage intake, even for just a few days, is the first step toward change. It brings awareness to what, why, and how much you are eating. It is the beginning stage to practicing mindfulness in eating.

As you become more mindful and deliberate with eating clean, whole foods, you will find yourself feeling good and energized, and you will have a more focused mind.

Staying upbeat and positive is easier because your physical body and mind feel good from eating good, clean food. You can't expect to be in a positive, optimistic, calm state of being if you are feeding your body junk. You can't expect to be in a positive, optimistic, calm state of being if you are not sleeping well. You can't expect to be in a positive, optimistic, calm state of being if you are not moving your physical body daily. Eat well, sleep well, move your body, and you will feel well. Feel well, and you will radiate a positive energy. Feel well, and you will think better. Think better, and you will act and speak better. Think, act, speak better, and you will change your life for the better, because you are radiating a positive energy. Do you see how every choice is connected and affects your physical body and how you feel?

Start adding more fruits and vegetables to your daily meal plan. Choose water as your beverage. Experiment with proteins. Journal your food intake. Eat slowly. Watch your portions. Pretty simple, yes?

Take a look at your food journal after one week. Do you nibble and snack too much? Are you eating too many processed foods? Are you drinking enough water? Do you eat your kid's food? Do you eat too late at night? Portions too large? Drinking too much alcohol? Eating too much animal protein? Eating too much sugar? Fast food? Eating out too much? Are you drinking too much caffeine? Not enough fruits and vegetables? Too many white carbs? Belly hurt after eating dairy? Feeling tired in the afternoon? Starving at the end of the day?

What will you tweak? Sometimes all it takes is to stop drinking your calories in the form of sugary drinks and choose to drink water instead to jumpstart you into healthy habits.

How about cutting out all "white" and processed foods?

Will you decide to manage your portions?

How about eating more fruits and vegetables so you don't have room for junk?

How about learning to cook more healthy meals?

The healthy choices are endless. Just start now. Small steps, small commitments, small tweaks. These small changes add up to huge benefits.

A Quick Note about Supplements

I am a firm believer in getting all your nourishment from good, clean healthy food. But, we do live in a world with toxins everywhere—from the food we eat, to the water we drink, and the air we breathe. So, it's a good thing to help your body out a bit with some good, purified, clean supplements.

I take wheat grass, vitamin D, omega-3, and a whole food multivitamin. This ensures that I am supporting my immune system, reducing inflammation in my body, and keeping my body healthy.

The supplement industry is not regulated, so I would make sure you go to a reputable organic market and talk to someone who is knowledgeable about supplements. Educate yourself. But don't get obsessed and crazy. Just make sure you're taking a purified brand (it should say it on the bottle for the omega-3's) and organic. Ask your doctor whether any supplements interfere with any medications you are taking. Or see a local naturopath MD.

I also have a love affair with my Vitamix blender. I love juicing and making nourishing smoothies. During the spring and summer, I make lots of juices and smoothies, which I call "nourishment in a glass." The abundance of in-season fruits and vegetables makes for nourishing drinks! Below are my top four steps to a nourishing juice or smoothie. This is such a quick way to get nourishment that it takes the excuse away of not having enough time for something healthy!

The first ingredient I choose is a healthy omega-3 fat. Again, the main thing you need to know about omega-3 fatty acid is that it is a natural anti-inflammatory for the body. Some of my top choices are walnuts, chia seeds, coconut milk, nut butter, or flaxseed. Always use a serving size!

The second ingredient is fruits and vegetables. Berries, kale, apples, bananas, and spinach are my top choices. Choose one or two ingredients for the fiber, antioxidants, vitamin, and mineral benefits!

The third ingredient I choose is a healthy protein. One scoop of whey protein or soy protein, one cup of Greek yogurt, or tofu are my top choices. Choose one!

The fourth ingredient is a nourishing add-in. Green tea powder, wheat grass powder, and Spirulina are my top choices. They are all filled with fiber, protein, antioxidants, vitamins, minerals, and an energy kick!

And last but not least, liquids. Water, coconut water, almond milk, and soy milk are my top choices.

When making smoothies or juices, go organic when possible. Honestly, I don't go too crazy with organic or nonorganic. Although organic is obviously the healthiest, cleanest choice, if you are practicing your other four fundamentals consistently every day, your body will naturally release toxins so a buildup doesn't happen and make you ill.

I also have a love affair with soups. I call my soup "nourishment in a pot." The basics ingredients are as follows: Sautee chopped onions, garlic, shitake mushrooms, carrots, and celery in a little olive oil for about eight minutes. Add three quarts of organic, low-sodium chicken broth, one can organic canned tomatoes, and one bag of previously soaked overnight beans (I usually use the variety package).

Bring to a boil and simmer until beans are cooked—about one hour and thirty minutes.

Add chopped organic kale and simmer for another ten minutes.

If using a lean protein, I usually sauté nitrate-free turkey sausage or organic cut-up chicken before adding the onions, garlic, etc. Enjoy nourishment in a pot!

Organic or not organic? I sometimes buy organic, sometimes not. I always buy the cleanest protein choices I can get, including grass-fed beef, organic chicken, and eggs. I cook a variety of seafood and fish. I do believe that if you are sweating every day and releasing the toxins out of your body, drinking enough water, and managing your state of mind and emotions, you can get away with not buying all organic. Although all organic or local is your cleanest and best way to keep pesticides off your plate, if you are engaging in all the other choose-well steps, you will be healthy. You can eat all organic, use all the cleanest and organic cleaning products, but if you are not moving and sweating and managing your emotions, it will be hard for your body to stay healthy. All these steps are directly connected to one another. I also hear complaints that organic is expensive. Well, you are going to pay one way or another if you don't take care of yourself. Sickness will cost you more.

I believe everyone can benefit from eating a high-fiber, clean diet and from helping the immune system out with supplements. However, for anyone with any disease or in any pain, I would suggest checking with your doctor or seeing a qualified nutritionist to get you personally on track with what is right for you individually.

Suggested Resources for Healthy Recipes

Eatingwell.com
Clean Eating magazine
Cookinglight.com

Fundamental Three:
Move it or Lose it

Ⅰf you don't use your body every day, you will lose it to disease, sickness, weakness, pain, and injury. A new study from Harvard suggests that inactivity can be as harmful to your health and well-being as smoking and that a sedentary lifestyle is the cause of one in ten deaths worldwide. That is an eye-opening statistic since it is totally preventable by choosing to get up off the coach and move! (Published online July 18, 2012, *The Lancet*.)

We are each blessed with 1,440 minutes per day. **You have thirty minutes to exercise at least four times per week. No "yeah but" excuses.** Sorry to be so blunt about this, but if you choose not to use thirty minutes four times per week to sweat, then you cannot be surprised with the result/consequence of that choice. If you don't use your body, you will lose it. That is the consequence of not exercising consistently.

As Hippocrates said, "That which is used develops, and that which is not used wastes away." Our bodies are meant to move. If you choose not to, and you accept excuses from yourself, the consequence of that choice is easy to see. Your body will get sick, and you will experience muscle and joint pain.

No exercise leads to a break down of the body. Muscles and bones atrophy and weaken. Toxins build up, and the heart, lungs, and organs start to deteriorate. The consequence? Illness, disease, and pain. You just won't feel well.

Suggested Attitude Practice: Shift your attitude from looking at exercise to "get skinny" to creating a fit, strong, and healthy body. It's all about keeping your body healthy so you can enjoy your life so much more. When your physical body is healthy, fit, and strong, you are able to handle life's challenges in a much more effective way, and you are able to enjoy all the pleasures in life in a much grander way. The health that you are experiencing is your creation, your responsibility, and your decision.

It baffles me sometimes to hear even my own relatives complain about their health when they are not doing what they need to do to take care of their body. How can you be surprised when illness, disease, and pain affect your body when you are not moving it or taking care of it? How can you complain about your illness or pain when you are not doing anything about it to help heal your body and get it stronger? Do you think just popping prescriptive drugs (with a list of side effects that pretty much says death) is the answer? Really? Just take a second a think about it. Studies have shown that reducing stress (managing your state of mind and emotions), eating well, and exercising reduce the risk of every known disease that ails man. Yet, we spend billions and billions of dollars on prescriptive drugs and get unhealthier and unhealthier. It just doesn't make sense.

If you are complaining about your health, stop. Start doing something about it to change it.

The Positive Consequences of a Regular Exercise Habit

You will feel good. Exercise releases "feel good" endorphins. Don't you want to walk through life feeling good, confident, strong, centered, clear-minded, and energized? Engage in some type of activity every day. Even if it is twenty minutes, and yes you have twenty minutes. Put the phone down, let Facebook be, and just move. You need to decide to make physical activity a priority. If you are using "no time" as your excuse for not exercising, then you have not made your health a priority to you. Make choices over a long period of time that support this decision about not making your health a priority, and your body will give you a wake-up call. It's not a matter of "if"; it is a matter of "when." According to a study by the *Journal of Sports and Exercise Psychology*, it takes just fifteen minutes of exercise to improve your mood. Just fifteen minutes! Peace and calmness are states of being that are easily practiced because you "moved" the stress out of your body and you feel good!

You will prevent disease. It is no secret at this point that exercise has been shown to reduce the risk of just about every single health problem known to man, from stroke to heart disease, to cancer and osteoporosis. Exercise not only strengthens your immune system, which is your body's natural defense against all kinds of illness and disease, sweating every day releases toxins out of your body. So sweat! Exercise also releases emotional stress and negativity from the body. You need to work stress out of your body, or it manifests as disease.

You will look fantastic. Although I would love to have you shift your focus to just being healthy, looking good is definitely a result of regular exercise. Exercise tones your body, improves your posture, makes your skin glow, and you will have more energy to enjoy your day. You will lose weight, and you will keep that weight off when you decide to exercise consistently. Exercise builds muscle tissue, which burns fat and prevents fat storage.

You will have less pain. Whether it is back pain, joint pain, or muscular pain, strengthening the muscles around your joints will reduce pain and overall aches.

Exercise makes you happy. Exercise has been shown to make you happy. Start your day with movement. It is very important to start your day feeling good. Since exercise makes you feel good, sweat in the morning. If the morning doesn't work for you, just do it as some particular point. If being happy is important to you, and I think it is for everyone, exercise.

What Kind of Exercise Do You Need Right Now?

When you ask yourself this question, what comes up as your answer? What is your body telling you it needs? Inside or outside? Class environment? Gentle or kick-butt type exercise? High intensity or low intensity? Dance or sport specific? Cardio? Strength? Is your back crying for core strength? What does your body need?

What I want to emphasize here is that **you need to listen to your body** and engage in an exercise program that is right for you and your lifestyle right here and right now. If your body is in pain, first analyze why you are in pain. There is always a cause, and the effect is pain. If you do too little exercise, and your body is weak, you will experience pain. If you do too much exercise, your body will tell you that you need to pull it back a bit. Pain is a signal to **stop** and analyze what is going on. Your body may be experiencing pain because of lots of emotional tension and stress, and a good aerobic workout is what you need, or sometimes pushing around some weights to get the tension out of your body is what you need. Sometimes if there is a lot of emotional stress going on, you may need yoga or Pilates and nothing too stressful on the body because your body is already experiencing emotional stress. So, pay attention.

I truly believe we need some type of movement daily. Our bodies are meant to move. If we don't, we feel tired, lethargic, and cranky. We lose muscle tone and strength, which causes all sorts of problems. Not to mention what happens when too much emotional tension is stored in the body. The consequence is always negative if you choose not to engage in physical activity. Don't allow yourself to get into a toxic cycle because you are not moving. Commit to doing some kind of movement every day, especially if you sit at a desk job. Think about it. You sleep, get up, sit in the car for your commute, sit at your desk all day, drive home sitting in your car, and then sit in front of the TV. Then we take a pill to try to alleviate any back pain we may have ... yikes.

If you are exhausted, ask yourself why. I know we are on the subject of exercise, but every choice you make affects everything in your life. Let's take feeling exhausted. Is it emotional? Is there something going on that you are trying to control and have no control over? Are you not exercising? Are you drinking too much caffeine and not enough water? Are you eating junk, which will make you feel exhausted? How are you sleeping? Here is the thing—as soon as you change **one** thing you can control, other changes start happening. If you start exercising to help your exhausted feeling, you will want to start eating better because your body will want to be nourished. You will also sleep better, because exercise helps you sleep. If you start meditating or praying to practice letting go, your body won't be holding on to emotional negativity, and you will feel at ease and not exhausted. If you have a headache, your body may need water. Or you may need to stand up and take a break from your desk. You may need some deep breathing, or you may need to listen to some music to release tension. Or you may need to take a walk or go for a run.

If you feel cranky, are you contemplating something or someone that makes you feel bad? Are you worrying? Is your mental state pretty negative? Maybe you need to strength train and work those negative feelings out of your body. Maybe you need to go out in nature to ground yourself and get some perspective. Maybe you need to sweat. Or go ahead and hit your "love" list and engage in something that will move attention away from feeling bad to feeling good.

What Do I Do and What Do I Teach?

Don't underestimate the power of taking a walk outside. One of my greatest joys is walking my dog, Christe, an hour a day. It's good for both mind and body. However, there are types of exercise that I recommend.

High-intensity training combined with core/weight training. This type of training prevents all sorts of disease, from heart disease to cancer. In my humble opinion, it is the most effect way to lose weight and keep it off, and improve fitness. It is what my outdoor boot camp is all about. Combining short bursts of high-intensity exercise with strength and core-training exercises is kick ass. If walking is your choice of exercise, you would alternate three or four minutes at a normal walking speed with one or two minutes at a brisk pace that is a bit uncomfortable for you. Add some strength-training moves such as walking lunges, squats, plyometrics, and pushups after a few interval bouts for huge calorie burning and to increase your metabolism. Raising and lowering your heart rate improves vascular function, burns a ton of calories, and makes the body more efficient at clearing fat and sugar from the blood.

Weight training. Weight training is the number-one way to increase your metabolism and increase your muscle strength around your joints. The benefits are endless. Free weights and body weight exercises are better for your body as far as increasing control, stability, and strength in the body.

Core workouts. A strong core will help you not only in sport-specific exercises like golf and tennis, but keeping a strong core will allow you to go through your daily life with ease, strength, and confidence. Pilates and core-specific exercises are a must to keep your back healthy, flexible, and strong.

Yoga/Pilates. It is a very calming type of workout that improves your core strength and flexibility and has been shown to reduce blood pressure. Breathing exercises and relaxation are important for managing stress, which is important for the health of your physical body and the health of your state of mind!

Total body non-impact exercise. The more muscles involved in an activity, the harder your body must work, and the stronger your body will be. Rowing, swimming, and cross-country skiing recruit muscles throughout the body without being too hard on the body.

Get outside. I can't stress enough how important it is to get outside. Hiking, walking, jogging—it is all good.

Find ways to be active all day. People who keep moving and are active all day in little ways—from taking stairs to parking the car far away from where you need to be, cleaning, gardening, etc.—burn more calories and are generally healthier than those who work out for thirty minutes and then sit at a computer all day. Just do your best to keep moving whenever and wherever possible.

What will enhance your chances of regularly engaging in physical activity?

- Be accountable to someone—a friend, trainer, workout buddy, etc.

- Choose an activity that you enjoy.

- Find a fitness center, outdoor boot camp class, or yoga/ Pilates studio near your office or home that makes it convenient to go to.

- Invest in some workout DVDs for training at home.

- Get outside and get some air. Tie your walking/running shoes on and just go. Wear a pedometer and aim for 10,000 steps per day. Just get up and go.

- Make the daily choice to get moving.

If you don't use your body, you can't be surprised when your body starts breaking down due to pain, injury, illness, or disease. If you don't use it, you lose it! No excuses, no justifications.

Do some type of movement everyday. You can always "do" something. Even a two-minute sun salutation gets your blood flowing. Everything counts. Fifteen minutes in the morning, fifteen minutes in the evening … it's all good. Break up your workouts. Whatever it takes to get you going and keep you consistent.

Practice patience. We live in a fast, quick-result society. Stick with whatever changes you are making for at least one month and then re-evaluate. Stay on track, never give up on yourself, and keep making healthy choices one day at a time. Your body is getting healthier after each workout you engage in. Just do your part and allow your body to its part.

If you are already exercising consistently—awesome! Is it challenging enough? Are you sweating every day? How is your flexibility? What does your body need right now? Do you need rest? Are you overtraining? Do you need to hire a professional to kick it up a notch?

Choose: What time of day will I work out? How much time? What days of the week? Class environment or at home? Outside or inside? What type of exercise?

Just get moving and never stop.

You always have the power of choice. Own it.

FUNDAMENTAL FOUR:
QUALITY ZZZ'S

QUALITY OF SLEEP, not so much the quantity, is so important for good health and the well-being of our body and state of mind.

When we deprive ourselves of a restful sleep, we notice the effect both mentally and physically almost immediately. In the short term, you may experience fatigue, irritability, increased stress, difficulty focusing, and careless mistakes. You may experience odd food cravings and over eat with sugar because your body is in need of energy. You probably won't have energy for your workouts, and that makes you feel even worse. Long-term effects include increased risk of more serious health problems, such as a weakened immune system, sluggish metabolism, diabetes, depression, obesity, and heart disease. Quality sleep is vital to our health.

How much is enough? Even though seven or eight hours a night is the recommended time, it is really individual, and you need to analyze what is right for you. Start with seven hours and see how you feel.

If you already know you are sleep deprived and experiencing the above symptoms, you need to start making choices that will help you get a better night's sleep. You are making it harder on yourself to manage your state of mind and emotions when you are exhausted. It is not easy to maintain a calm, optimistic, and at-ease attitude when you are tired. Monitor how much sleep you are getting, how your mood and energy level is throughout the day, and start tweaking what you can. To stay focused, think clearly, and make deliberate choices, you must be well rested. Journal how much sleep you are getting, and how you feel. What is good for one person is not necessarily enough for another. Remember, it is quality not quantity. Write down how many hours of sleep you get, what your evening ritual is, what time you eat and what you eat, whether you exercised that day, what you drank throughout the day, and how your mood and attitude was that day.

Tips for Better Quality Sleep

- Try to rise out of bed at the same time each day, and go to bed the same time each day. This regulates your body's inner clock.
- Make sure your room is dark, quiet, and comfortable.
- Avoid alcohol before bed.
- Shut down from all mental stimulation during the hour before bed. No phones, no computers, no TV, no work, etc. Totally unplug from all input.
- Never watch the news before bed. Planting bad news into your mind before you go to sleep is never a nourishing, uplifting, and helpful choice.
- Get exercise during the day. Exercise helps you sleep better!
- Avoid smoking, caffeine, or any type of stimulant two hours before bed.
- Give your body two hours to digest any food eaten at night before falling to sleep. Try to eat an evening meal that contains tryptophan. This sleep-inducing amino acid is found in turkey, chicken, fish, soybeans, nuts, and cheese.
- Eat light at night.
- Try not to drink too many liquids at night. Getting up to go to the bathroom frequently interrupts your sleep. Get most of your water during the day.
- Never replay all that went wrong during the day or all that you are worried or fearful about. Never contemplate a situation you are angry, upset, or anxious about.
- Pray.
- Meditate.
- Mentally visualize all the good in your life, and say, "Thank you, God." Plant goodness in your mind before falling to sleep.

- Take a warm bath infused with some essential relaxing oils (such as lavender and chamomile along with two cups of Epsom salt).
- Read inspiring books.
- Enjoy intimacy and sex with your partner.
- Listen to soothing music.
- Do some light stretching or yoga moves while breathing deeply.
- Do some deep breathing and affirm, "All is well, and my life is unfolding as it should," as you fall asleep. Or use any other calming, nourishing, comforting affirmation with your deep breathing.
- Visualize goodness before you sleep; never contemplate your problems.
- Monitor your sleep. Do you know how much sleep you need in order to feel rested? What habits do you need to stop in order to get quality sleep? What do you need to start doing to get a quality sleep?

You always have the power of choice. Own it.

FUNDAMENTAL FIVE:
STAY HYDRATED

THE IMPORTANCE OF drinking water and staying hydrated should not be underestimated. How much water are you drinking right now? If you are not in the habit of drinking water, I strongly suggest you put your attention on increasing your intake until you regularly are taking in at least eight cups a day. Now, I know this is the recommended amount, and it is a good starting point to analyze how much water you need to feel well.

I am talking about clear, fresh water. Not artificially flavored water, not diet anything, not calorie-free anything. Just pure, fresh water.

Think about this for a second. Our bodies are made up of at least 60 percent water. Since we are made up of mostly water, what do you think the consequence of not drinking enough is? You may be feeling your body's thirst already.

Chronic dehydration, which is probably affecting most of us today, has been shown to be a huge contributor to illness and disease. Just think about this. It has been documented that: our blood is 83 percent water; our muscles are 75 percent water; our brain is 70 percent water; our bones are 22 percent water; our lungs are 90 percent water.

Now, given these percentages, what do you think the consequence is of not taking in enough water? Here are a few: Toxins building up in the blood, causing illness and disease; foggy and unclear thinking; fatigue and irritability; muscle cramps; asthmatic conditions; migraines and headaches; constipation; dry mouth; infrequent urination and urine that is darker in color than usual.

If you are experiencing any of the dehydration symptoms, drink your water! Before you pop an over-the-counter med for a headache or muscle cramp, hydrate!

Some schools of thought believe drinking tea and eating soups and lots of fruits and vegetables that contain lots of water don't really count in proper hydration. I tend to believe that these foods are hydrating, but I would still aim for the eight glasses. You may find yourself needing more, especially in the summer months and when you are sweating a lot when working out. Try to drink most of your water during the day so your sleep is not interrupted during the evening.

Be aware of the calories you are drinking. Being careful about what you are drinking when it's not water is a very healthy practice to get into. Specialty coffee drinks are heavy with sugary syrups and pack in calories. A better choice would be plain coffee with a little milk, or even better, antioxidant rich green tea. During the summer months, watch the pina coladas and margaritas. These drinks not only spike your blood-sugar level, they pack in a good 800 calories in one drink. Scary. Choose a glass of red wine or light beer. Let's talk about soda. Yikes. It has absolutely no nutritional value whatsoever, and don't even think that diet soda is better. If you have a soda habit, make an effort to break it. You can do it. Juice drinks are another sugar-laden, no-nutritional-value drink. Choose to eat the real fruit (apple, oranges) instead of the juice. You will be getting nourishing fiber along with the natural sugars that are in the fruit. If you do buy juice, make sure it is 100 percent juice with no added sugar. Try diluting the juice with water to lessen the sugar content.

Suggested Practice: Start right now and aim for eight glasses of pure, fresh water per day. Get into the habit of drinking two cups when you get up in the morning and a half hour before you eat your meal to get your digestive system ready for food. Even if you are (hopefully) eating plenty of fruits and vegetables, soups, and herbal teas, I would still aim for eight glasses of water per day. The consequences of chronic dehydration are toxic to the body. You just won't feel well if you don't drink enough water. And if you don't feel well, again, it's hard to stay in a positive, optimistic frame of mind.

Always keep water on hand. Sipping it throughout the day will help prevent dehydration. Eat lots of fruits and veggies, and when drinking alcohol, always drink water to prevent dehydration!

It is such a simple, small change with huge, positive effects, and yet most of us are walking around totally dehydrated. Amazing.

One of the most fascinating things about water comes from the research of Masaru Emoto, who documented the effect of negative feelings on water in his book called *The Hidden Messages in Water*. In a nutshell, he showed the amazing structural changes in water when given good, positive, loving feeling and words; the water was crystal clear, brilliant, and clean. When the water was given negative vibes through feeling and words, the water became dirty and toxic. That is huge. Imagine what the positive and negative feelings are doing to your body since your body is made up of mostly water. That's another reason to monitor yourself at all times and consciously shift yourself away from negative feelings and vibes.

Recommended Reading:
Your Body's Many Cries for Water
The Hidden Messages in Water

You always have the power of choice. Own it.

CONCLUSION

S O, THERE YOU have it—the five simple fundamentals to a fit, strong, healthy body and state of mind. Where do you start? What do you do? There are many ways to implement this lifestyle.

1. You can go back and take a look at your answers to the lifestyle questions and start implementing the action choice and state of being choice you personally made and go from there. Stick with your practice for one month. After one month, answer the questions again and celebrate the healthy changes you have made! Move forward tweaking, adjusting and choosing well!

2. Pick one *Choose Well to Live Well* steps to manage your state of mind and emotions, and choose one other fundamental to implement. Practice for four weeks. For example, you might start a meditation practice and start drinking more water for four weeks. Or you may start a blessings-consciousness practice as you start eating clean for four weeks. Maybe you will start practicing optimism as you start exercising consistently. Whatever you choose, just be patient and stay persistent and enjoy your journey! Keep choosing and tweaking until you are living all five fundamentals as a personal lifestyle.

If the concepts in this book have opened your eyes to, at the very least , pay more attention to what you are choosing in the way you think, speak, and behave, then I am thrilled beyond what I can express. With awareness comes positive change.

Stay in the driver's seat of your health and well-being, and only good will come from it!

Never give your power to choose to any circumstance or any person. **You always have a choice**. You can always **do** something to make your life and state of health better, and you can always **be** someone better than you were yesterday. Own it.

You only have one day at a time to live, so live it and choose well!

Please visit www.choosewelltolivewell.com for more support in living the Choose Well lifestyle!

If you are facing in the right direction,
all you need to do is keep on walking.
—Buddhist Proverb

This book is intended to help you with basics on what it takes to be healthy, fit, and strong in both mind and body. It is made up of the practices I personally live and teach my clients on a daily basis. Please seek professional help when needed. I am not a doctor, nor do I claim to be. I am a licensed health and wellness coach, certified personal trainer, certified Adventure Boot camp trainer, and a licensed massage therapist who is very passionate about helping people live healthy, fit, and happy lives! As you practice your fundamentals daily, enjoy and embrace all that you experience. The universe will provide people, situations, and circumstances that come to you for a purpose and experience. You will find yourself in awe of the unfolding of your life. Enjoy.

Thank you for allowing me to be a part of your health and wellness journey!

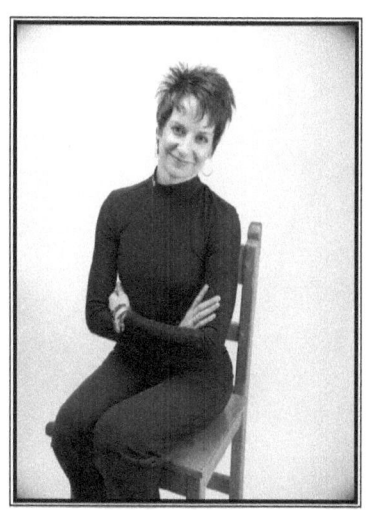